CLEANSE YOUR BLOOD

The Complete No-Nonsense Guide to Reversing Diabetes, Prediabetes & Metabolic Syndrome

By Drew Coster MS

Copyright © 2019 by **Drew Coster**

All rights reserved. No part of this publication may be reproduced, distributed or transmitted in any form or by any means, without prior written permission.

Disclaimer: The information provided in this book is designed to provide helpful information on the subjects discussed and is not a substitute for the medical advice of physicians. Please regularly consult a physician in matters relating to your health, especially where diagnosis or medical attention is required. The publisher and author are not responsible for any specific health needs that may require medical supervision and are not liable for any damages or negative consequences from any treatment, action, application or preparation, to any person reading or following the information in this book.

Cleanse Your Blood: The Complete No-Nonsense Guide to Reversing Diabetes, Prediabetes, & Metabolic Syndrome

Acknowledgments

I'd first like to thank my wonderful wife for supporting me in writing this book. I'm eternally grateful for every draft you read, suggested edits, and basically for just putting up with me all these years. Without you, this wouldn't have been possible, and I love you to bits.

I'd also like to say a huge thank you to Dr. Rosemary Ku for believing in me and teaching me so much about chronic disease. You're an amazing human and one of the few doctors who really understands what it takes to treat chronic disease in ways that don't just revolve around medication. The medical field needs more people like you, and I appreciate your support, comments and participation in this book more than I can say.

And finally, I'd like to dedicate this book to my mother and father who died way too soon from chronic disease.

Foreword

Millions of people worldwide are getting sick with type 2 diabetes, prediabetes, and metabolic syndrome. When left untreated, these conditions progress to life-threatening conditions such as heart disease, kidney failure, stroke, dementia, and even cancer. Unlike diseases that spread by pathogens such as viruses, bacteria, or parasites; these conditions spread through something much more insidious - an unhealthy lifestyle. Chronic stress, poor sleep, sedentary habits, and unhealthy food choices are inescapable in modern life so even if you are healthy today, you may still be at risk in the near future.

As daunting as this is, understanding the root cause provides hope for how to reverse these conditions. With consistent improvements in lifestyle based on the latest metabolic research; medications may no longer be necessary, energy levels will soar, and you can add many vibrant years to your life. It all starts with one tiny behavior at a time, right now.

As a physician, I'm sad to say that many healthcare systems unfortunately are not equipped to support people through the process of lifestyle change. Many providers are not properly trained in this area and are often skeptical that patients can make dramatic improvements in their health. As a result, many patients with chronic conditions are reflexively put on medications without diving into the reasons why they have the disease and what they can do about it.

Anyone who has ever been told "Eat less. Exercise more." knows this is not an effective prescription. While you should listen to your physician's advice, it's important to educate yourself and understand that it may be possible to reverse your condition. Ask your physician questions about what you learn and help them be a part of your journey.

Time and time again, I've seen patients with chronic conditions experience jarring wake-up calls. Some find themselves on the verge of losing their eyesight or kidney function due to diabetes or their loved one had a debilitating stroke as a result of years of hypertension. Once reminded of what's at stake if they don't change, these patients are willing to do whatever it takes to get back to good health and many succeed. These success stories may not be the majority yet, but I believe they could be.

In *Cleanse Your Blood*, Drew has provided a blueprint for how to completely turn around your health. This book isn't a fad diet or exercise plan. Instead, it will encourage you to take a closer look at what you are doing today, the causes and effects of your behaviors, and how you can improve not just your health but also overall well-being. Armed with the latest science, humor, humility, and a profound understanding of lifestyle change; Drew's guidance empowers everyone from all walks of life. His one-on-one work as a psychotherapist and health coach has saved countless lives and now, he's sharing his insights with you.

This book is for you if you've been diagnosed with diabetes, prediabetes, or metabolic syndrome but were never told you had a choice to change your fate. This book is for you if you love someone with these conditions so that you can provide hope and support throughout the journey back to health. And this book is for you if you have ever worried about developing these diseases. It's never too late or early to take control over your health.

Rosemary Ku, MD/MBA/MPH

CONTENTS

The Journey Begins 1
MIND WORK 5
Preparing to Change 6
Approach to Change 9
The Cycle of Change 20
Building Your Team 27
Creating A Benefits List 32
Potential Fears and Challenges 37
Potential Obstacles 42
Recognize Emotional Eating 46
Managing Trigger Foods 52
Exception Eating 60
Self-Care Action Plan 63
Weekly Action Plan 69
The First Two Weeks 71
Maintenance Eating 76
Going Forward 79
FIVE PILLARS 80
Five Pillars of Good Health 81
Pillar #1: Sleep 85
Pillar #2: Water 106
Pillar #3: Nutrition 117
Pillar #4: Stress 130
Pillar #5: Exercise 140
NUTRITION 150
Nutrition Made Simple 151

Portion Sizes 154
Meal Timing 157
Food Choices 162
Two Week Meal Plan 183
Substitutes for Your Favorite Foods 198
Understanding Nutrition Labels 210
YOUR BLOOD 224
Understanding Your Blood 225
What is Insulin? 235
What's Happening to Your Hormones? 240
Your Blood Work 248
The Spread of Poor Blood Health 272
QUESTIONS 287
FAQ 288
You've Got This! 300
References 301

The Journey Begins

The first thing I want to do is reassure you diabetes, prediabetes, and metabolic syndrome are not life sentences. I know this because I've helped many people like you change their unhealthy blood to healthy within a short time. From working with talented doctors on the cutting edge of chronic disease, I have the knowledge and experience to help you reverse your condition. All I ask is you read this book with an open mind and a willingness to cleanse your blood for good. If you do that, then I know you will be successful in reversing your condition with little trouble.

As a psychotherapist I'm interested in helping people understand their process of change. And one of my main goals is to help you understand yours rather than just tell you what to do. This approach will be valuable not just for cleansing your blood, but all aspects of your life. I believe the more awareness you have about how you approach change, the more benefits you'll gain in all aspects of your life. Prescribing a one-size-fits-all approach is a short-term, short-sighted approach and not one that will help you be successful.

Books on your blood condition often focus on food as the main problem *and* solution to reversing your condition. But the reality is food is only one part of the whole story. What will help you more is learning how to balance multiple aspects of your lifestyle. I call these aspects the Five Pillars of Good Health. And understanding how these Pillars work together will make reversing your condition far easier than just focusing on one aspect like food.

In truth, even though all three conditions: diabetes, prediabetes and metabolic syndrome have different names, the way to reverse them all is practically the same. And because of that, all the information contained in this book is going to be relevant for all three conditions, no matter if you've just been diagnosed with metabolic syndrome or if you've had diabetes for many years. If you follow the information contained in this book closely, I promise you'll soon have all the knowledge you need to cleanse your blood, no matter where your starting point.

To that end, I've split this book into five sections, with each offering insight into the process of cleansing your blood. These sections are Mind Work, Five Pillars of Good Health, Nutrition, Your Blood and Questions.

Mind Work will help you understand the change process and how you approach change. The exercises in this section will encourage you to consider your motivation; spot unhelpful negative thinking; tackle emotional eating; and how to create a space for self-care. This is where the work you do now will build a stronger foundation for later. This section is especially valuable if you've ever tried to diet or cleanse your blood before and things just didn't work out. And for those who haven't engaged in any self-reflection in the past, you might find this section very enlightening.

The Five Pillars section will show you why balancing different facets of your life is important. Here I'll explain why focusing on one aspect of health rather than the collective whole is not a suitable path to long-term health. Sometimes you don't have to change everything to be healthy, but we do need to change the right things.

The **Nutrition** section will breakdown the foods which will help cleanse your blood the most, and the ones that are best avoided or kept as treats. You might feel tempted to jump straight to this section, however, I encourage you to continue through the **Mind Work** section first. Making an effective action plan, and understanding any emotional or cognitive roadblocks you have, will serve you more in the long-run than just eating differently.

Your Blood section is going to explain to you what's going on in your body and why your condition is more about hormone dysfunction than just high blood sugar. I will also help you decipher what your blood test result are really saying.

Finally, in the **Questions** section I'll answer the most common questions I've been asked which might also apply to you. At the end of this book if you have a question which I haven't covered, then email me at cleanseyourblood@drewcoster.com and I will do my best to answer.

Thanks for reading and let's go get your blood healthy.

PART ONE:

MIND WORK

*"Give a man a fish and you feed him for a day;
teach a man to fish and you feed him for a lifetime."*
- Maimonides

Preparing to Change

Talking about change is easy but doing it can be hard. Lifestyle change can be a challenge because we get comfortable with how things are, even if those things are not good for us. If you're reading this book because you have either diabetes, prediabetes or metabolic syndrome then you know at this point in your life you need to cleanse your blood. But how do you do that?

In my experience, approaching change with a 'I'll see how it goes' attitude will not cut it. Knowing what you will do, and how you will approach that change will give you the best opportunity for success. Which is why I want to share some techniques and exercises I know will help you reverse your condition using Cognitive Behavior Therapy (CBT) techniques and little sprinkle of theory to help you understand how your brain might be making change hard for you.

The exciting part about the journey ahead is that it's in your hands. You get to make the decisions that will affect your life and your blood because nobody else can do this for you. By owning this journey, you will be empowering yourself to change, and that's way better than being told what to do or just being given medication, which won't solve your problem.

In my therapeutic experience, if you don't have ownership and a clear understanding on why change is important to you, then challenging any entrenched habits you have can be tough, if not impossible. Not because you don't want to change unhealthy habits or certain aspects of yourself, but more likely you have habits that are so stubborn they will fight you. We all have that sneaky inner voice who undermines our decisions. I'm sure you know the one, that inner saboteur who whispers in your ear: "It's only one small piece of cake, it won't hurt? Go on, eat it." Trust me, we all have one.

You might have experienced this inner saboteur if you've tried giving up an unhealthy habit before but found you quit soon after making the decision to change. Like making a New Year's resolution to go the gym every day but ended up paying a year's membership and never showing up. Or vowing never to eat chocolate cake again, but then gave in the next time someone puts a slice in front of you. This struggle is real and makes lasting change seem difficult.

Because I understand this inner voice and what motivates people to change, I've approached this book in a way that teaches you how to change, before you tackle actual change. I do think learning how to change is more important than the practical tasks of change, because anyone can follow a diet or exercise plan given to them but is that plan suitable for you and your lifestyle? You might have many challenges that others don't have. You may have a harsh inner critic and saboteur who you need to learn to quiet before you become successful. Just filling your shopping cart with organic superfoods (which probably won't make the slightest difference) because somebody told you that was the only way to cleanse your blood, won't help most people.

If you need to cleanse your blood, then I think you need a good roadmap before you start, which is why I will help you plan a successful path to change, while uncovering your inner motivation to change. By going through the exercises in the book, together we'll build a robust roadmap which you can refer to anytime you feel stuck, bored, or disillusioned with how things are going.

And if making plans and lists is not your thing and you want to skip ahead, I respect that, but I would advise against it. I do believe when it comes to changing lifestyle habits for good, we all need to slow down, understand the direction we need to go; be clear on why we are looking to change and then follow through with an informed process.

The truth is, you know yourself far more than I can know you. But even then, do you really know what's going on in your head when it comes to change?

To keep us on the same page and working towards cleansing your blood I've include worksheet throughout, which might be helpful to you. These worksheets are all free to download from my website drewcoster.com/worksheets

In this section you will learn how to:
- Think about how you approach change
- Understand how change works.
- Create a benefits list for your journey.
- Understand your emotional and thinking roadblocks.
- Get to grips with your relationship with food.
- Navigate the first two weeks.

My promise to you, is that I will impart all the knowledge I have on cleansing your blood in a simple step-by-step way. And at the end, you'll have the right mindset and tools to be healthy for the rest of your life. And that is something worth doing.

Approach to Change

How much do you know about yourself and how you approach change? Are you the person who is gung-ho and rushes into change, or are you more cautious and thoughtful about the process? Gaining insight into our own emotional roadblocks and unhelpful thoughts can be extremely helpful when we change something as important as our health. The insights you'll gain by working through this section will highlight your strengths and weaknesses to the change process.

To help you gain more self-awareness in your approach to change, I'd like to offer you a simple questionnaire. There are no right answers, nor will there be a scientific breakdown of your score. What I'm encouraging is curiosity about how you approach change. Your answers can be as brief as you like but writing something can be valuable for gaining self-awareness.

Your Change Questionnaire

1. Are you making this change for you, or because someone else suggested it?
2. How long have you been thinking of reversing your blood condition?
3. Have you taken action before to cleanse your blood? And if you did, how long did it take before you gave up or tried something else?
4. Do you engage in negative self-talk if things don't go right?
5. How do you respond when you don't see progress?
6. Would you give up your favorite foods if you knew they were part of the problem with your blood condition?

7. If I told you it could take a year of constant lifestyle change for your blood to reach healthy levels, would you continue?
8. Are you open to new ideas to reverse your condition even if those ideas don't align with your current understanding of diabetes, prediabetes or metabolic syndrome?
9. Would you say you're more disciplined or spontaneous with life choices?

Gaining insight into potential sticking points will be helpful over the coming pages. We all understand success breeds success. Even if you've struggled with change before, this time you'll overcome any roadblocks you have because you will be more prepared. Go through each stage and be open with yourself. Build the most robust plan you can, because the one thing a book can't do for you is make the choices you'll need to cleanse your blood. As much as I wish I could be there in person to guide you through this process, I'm not. You are the leader of this expedition, and all I can do is help you create a path that will lead you to the top of your mountain.

If I had one mantra to impart for this entire process it would be this: Be consistent and strive for progress rather than perfection.

Consistency is Key

There will be times when the choices you make aren't as good as you'd like, and that's okay. That's being human. But what will aid you more than anything as you build your program to cleanse your blood, is to be as consistent as possible in thought and action. If you constantly dip in and out of cleansing your blood, through poor choices and lack of consistency, you won't see the results you desire. This inconsistency can lead to frustration, which might lead you to abandon your program.

I've seen how successful people can be when they are consistent with my guidelines. However, consistent doesn't mean rigid. I don't subscribe to the rigid approach to change. Too often, rigidity breeds contempt and boredom and that's no fun for anyone. Being strict for a few days or weeks can be helpful to get you in the groove of change, but long-term rigidity will sap all the enjoyment of the process.

There are many reasons for being consistent, but the main one is to create new healthy habits over a long-time. For if we are consistent with a choice, and repeat it over and over, we can retrain our brain more successfully. By doing this we are replacing those old habits which aren't supportive of our health anymore. Ultimately, our long-term success will come from challenging and replacing these old habits and I'll talk more about that later in the Cycle of Change. Consistency really is key and before you know it, you'll be in a healthy routine, not even thinking about what you need to do to cleanse your blood.

Progress Not Perfection

Those who followed my guidance with an open mind and a realistic approach tend to do better than those who demand perfection. Rolling with the ups-and-downs of change teaches us valuable lessons about progress. Because even the smallest change becomes a win.

The problem with perfectionist thinking is what happens when things don't go to plan. Holding such an extreme mindset often leads to frustration if each week isn't better than the last. This frustration spreading like a virus until they abandon their program. Not because the program didn't work, but because their thinking couldn't withstand the complexity of human inconsistency.

Which is why I advocate progress not perfection from the very beginning.

The race to do everything perfectly can rob us of the learning experiences we gain from failing. And it doesn't matter how many of the Five Pillars of Good Health you need to balance (more on that soon), if you attack this journey with the attitude of being perfect, it will be a long and frustrating journey.

Over the next few pages I'll talk about the Cycle of Change, and why failing and relapse are all part of healthy change. Knowing you will screw up and make mistakes is part of becoming healthy and embracing that idea will empower you to stay consistent and keep working towards healthy blood.

Perfection is an ideal. A shining beacon we can marvel at, but it isn't helpful when dealing with humans. You will have many successes on this journey and some failures. Some days will be good, others frustrating. That's because life is complex. It doesn't bend to our will. But progress over time will lead to success. It's that simple.

Thinking Traps

Over the coming weeks there will be plenty of obstacles coming your way. We'll address more of the physical ones soon but first I want to introduce you to how our own thinking can be the main saboteur in our quest for better health.

Thinking traps are the common thoughts we have about ourselves, life and the world that can hold us back if we let them. Thinking traps are also known as cognitive distortions because these thoughts distort how we look at our world. You may not be aware of it, but we all have an inner blueprint we follow, our guide to staying safe in the world. Well, thinking traps play a large part in how healthy our blueprint is because if we get stuck in certain traps then it will distort how we perceive our reality. These traps don't have to be debilitating to be unhelpful. If we are unaware, we're engaging in unhealthy Thinking Traps we are destined to repeat them, over and over. This can then diminish our ability to stick to a change plan or to see the world in a different way.

What makes these traps so unhealthy is they also trigger how we feel and behave. And these feelings and behaviors then trigger how we think. We can get stuck in a vicious circle of negative thinking with the self-perpetuating thinking-feeling-behaving.

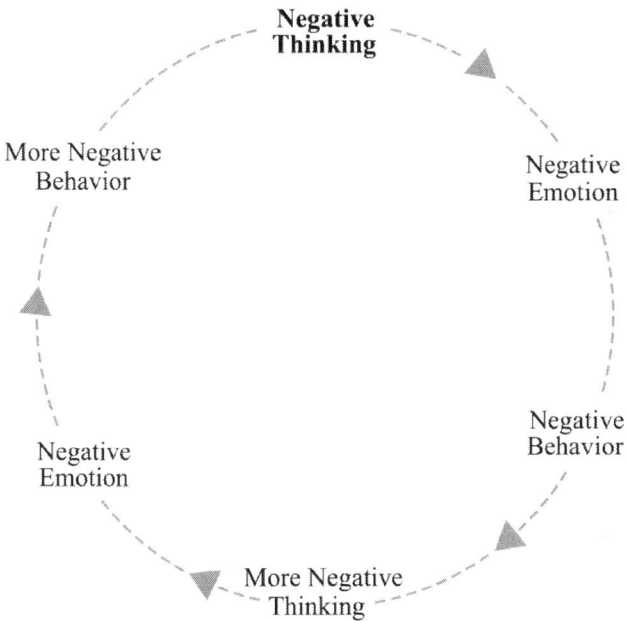

What this image shows is how easy it is to get stuck in a negative rut with our thinking. Don't feel bad if you recognize yourself doing any of the following thinking traps because to differing degrees, we all fall into them. Most are minor traps and can be overcome. However, sometimes these traps lead to extreme negative thinking, which brings us back to the vicious cycle of negative thinking. If you find you tend to think in extremes, I highly recommend you work with a CBT therapist to counter these traps.

One of the most important things about changing our thinking traps is learning to stop the thoughts. In the beginning this isn't easy, but in time you'll get used to hearing the trap words you are using and stopping yourself. One of the simplest methods is to learn the STOP! method. This is when you say out loud, Stop! when you catch yourself using any of the following traps. This might sound ridiculous, and it might feel that way in the beginning, but as soon as you learn how to catch your thinking traps, you'll be far clearer in your thinking. If you don't have confidence saying Stop! out loud, then say it in your mind. But when you do, also imagine a stop sign or a red traffic light to give the thought some added emphasis.

In CBT there are around sixteen thinking traps, but I'll highlight the six most common associated with the change process. Becoming aware of these traps and changing how we think, is a great first step towards self-care and breaking old habits.

All-or-Nothing Thinking

This trap is also known as black-and-white thinking, because it is about having thoughts that lie on the ends of a spectrum. With all-or-nothing thinking there is no gray area. Things are right or wrong; good or bad; win or fail. This also ties into perfectionism and can derail good progress.

Often these Thinking Traps lead people to abandon their journey to wellness after the first mistake. You might be this person or know someone like this? Often this thinking trap will lead a person to give up on the change process early because of the faulty thinking if things don't go right from the beginning. The thinking will tend to lead to: things bad = I failed. And when they fail, they might as well just give up - all-or-nothing.

This is the most common trap for people who are hard on themselves. The trouble is, having slips, trips and falls on your way to reversing your condition is very healthy, but this thinking trap won't let someone accept that reality.

All-or-nothing thinking is the worst trap to fall into if you want long-term success. Therefore, I go back to the mantra: Progress not perfection. It's okay to trip and make mistakes. It's normal to not eat well all the time, or not go to bed at a reasonable hour or get stressed at work. These things happen, and when they do, learn to accept them.

All-Or-Northing Example

Thought: I shouldn't have had that chocolate bar, I've ruined everything. I'm such a loser. Now, I must start all over again.
Triggered Emotion: Depression, anger, guilt and self-loathing.
Triggered Behavior: Sabotage eating and self-punishment.

Solution to All-or-Nothing Thinking:

Repeat this rational thought daily: It's okay to be fallible. I'm human and one slip doesn't mean I've failed. Instead I will continue with my progress and learn to accept these slips.

Having a counter thought to all these traps is important. Once you recognize you are falling into the trap, just stop yourself and address your thought with rational adult thinking. This might sound simplistic, but learning to counter irrational, unhelpful thinking is a big part of learning to rewrite our internal blueprint and overcome old habits. The main problem we all have with our blueprint is that it was created when we were children. And a lot of the thoughts and beliefs we hold are based on child-like thinking. Letting a child's thinking run your life is not good when we become adults, which is why we need to counter any thinking trap with a more realistic, adult thoughts.

At first, the Solution Thought might not 'feel' right, and that's okay. Keep going. Like any mantra, repetition helps give it strength. Keep working to counter your thinking traps and in time, you'll accept the truth in it and find more middle ground in your thinking.

Emotional Reasoning

Because so much of our thinking influences how we feel, this trap is important to understand when we are working to reverse a physical condition. Based on the premise we accept our feelings as truth, Emotional Reasoning is often driving faulty conclusions. For example, when you begin the journey to cleanse your blood, you might be changing old eating habits which means you begin eating healthily. But when we give up certain foods, we can feel more tired than normal for a while. You might get headaches, or a cold which can lead to a low mood. These symptoms are quite typical when we remove sugar from our diet (I'll talk more about this later) but because we feel down or depressed, our emotional reasoning trap kicks in and we conclude: I feel bad, so the plan isn't working (and then maybe we'll add an extra kick in the backside), therefore I've failed.

This negative emotional reasoning then feeds other traps into another vicious cycle. This negative thinking drives our unhealthy emotions, which drives our unhelpful behavior over and over again. Just from faulty emotional reasoning we conclude we have failed because we *feel* bad. Feelings are not thoughts!

Solution to Emotional Reasoning:

Learn to assess a situation by asking questions of yourself:

- "Just because I feel down, does that mean I've failed?"
- "Am I jumping to conclusions because I feel a strong emotion?"
- "Where is the evidence to back-up how I think about this situation?"

Try to step out of your feelings and learn to see if you have patterns of emotional reasoning which you use to jump to conclusions based on your mood.

Labeling

Criticize ourselves and our behavior is very common, but sometimes we can take it too far. Labeling is when that voice in your head is always putting you down, calling you a 'loser' or 'hopeless' or a 'failure'. These labels are too extreme and far to unfair. As a human you are too complex to be boiled down into one label. Even if you mess up, trip and don't do your best, you are still not a loser. You are a complex human being who sometimes makes a mistake.

When you call yourself a name, learn to Stop! and correct yourself. Again, these types of labels come from a child place. Children make these simple connections because they cannot understand the nuance and complexity of life. In a child mind, things are right or wrong. Which means you are either good or bad. Don't let that old thinking derail you from your journey to better health. Be kinder to yourself.

Solution to Labeling:

"I'm such an idiot" – "No, I'm not an idiot. I made a mistake, people do. I'll learn from this and move on."

Overgeneralizing

Words such as 'always', 'never' or 'ever'' are absolutes. When we use these words, we are putting up barriers to our success because we are thinking something is always this way, when in truth, they are not. We say things like, "*I always fail at sticking to things. I'll never reverse my diabetes.*" These types of absolutes are irrational and tie in with another thinking trap, all-or-nothing thinking.

Overgeneralizing often takes a situation that is a problem and overgeneralizes to the point it becomes like the end of the world an unrealistic. This overgeneralizing often ties into how children make conclusions; if they experience a setback, it is very common to hear them say: "*I'll never do this right!*" Then, as we grow-up and we hit setbacks, we automatically overgeneralize and tell ourselves we'll 'never do this' or 'I always screw-up'. Even though we know that isn't true, saying the words gives it power in our mind and this is what becomes self-limiting. Why bother trying to change if your brain is telling you: "*You'll never change.*"

Solution to Overgeneralizing:

When you catch yourself using these absolutes, Stop! Access your adult voice and let the child thinking know this isn't true – "*I can reverse my condition. It might take me time and there might be setbacks but saying I will never do it is plain wrong. I have completed many things in my life, and this will be no exception.*"

Should-ing

The tyranny of Shoulds is often a rigid command that can leave us feeling anxious and depressed. Should-ing is often a prefix to all the other traps in this list, adding an extra layer of condemnation to our thinking. If we live a life based on Should-ing we'll never feel satisfied.

There are two main types of Should-ing which can cause a problem. The first is Reflective Shoulds. These are the type of Shoulds we use when reflecting on a past situations. Telling ourselves what we should have done better: "*I shouldn't have had that slice of cake. I'm such a loser.*"

The other critical should is Rule Should-ing. These are Shoulds we've internalized when growing up and are usually based on rigid rules others have taught us: "*I shouldn't question my doctor. I should just get on with it and do as she says.*"

Should-ing creates an internal push-pull conflict that can cause paralysis to success. If we're constantly reflecting on what we didn't do and what we should have done, then it's possible to become depressed because in hindsight, you can do everything better. If we live a life of Rule Should-ing, we'll live a life of anxiety because we'll often run into rules, we don't believe in, but disobeying these rules will cause inner turmoil: "*I should always be perfect.*"

One last note on Should-ing. There are also some Shoulds that are realistic and not rigid. These are generally harmless and don't need attention. They come in the form of recommendations such as: "*You should go see that new movie, it's great.*" "*You should take a coat, it will rain later.*"

Solution to Should-ing:

Use the Stop! strategy and ask yourself if this should is helpful or not.

Rigid Should: "*I should be perfect.*" -- Stop! – "*Being perfect is impossible. I'd like to get things right and do well, but I know I'll sometimes get things wrong. I don't like that idea, but it's realistic and I'll be okay.*"

Reflective Should: "*I shouldn't have had that slice of cake. I'm such a loser.*" -- Stop! – "*It would have been better if I didn't have that slice of cake, but I did. I'm not happy about my choice but next time I'll do better at saying no. It's not the end of the world.*"

Realistic Should: *"I should take an umbrella as it's raining."* -- Stop! – *"Yeah, that might be a good idea."*

The Cycle of Change

Now you know some of the thinking traps you might fall into, the next step towards change is understanding the process. I'd like to show you something I know is effective. Changing habits can be difficult because we have that blueprint inside of us that I mentioned in the last section. This blueprint informs how we think, what we believe and how to approach certain situations. Created throughout our formative years, our blueprint is an amalgamation of all our opinions, experiences, likes, and dislikes.

This blueprint is like our map of how to live in the world, but it doesn't mean anytime we try and deviate from this map and do something unfamiliar, we will struggle. Imagine your blueprint is like Google maps. When you follow the maps instruction on how to get to a destination, things are straightforward - turn left, turn right, exit here. But when you choose a road that isn't on the route, Google will keep re-routing to get you back towards your original destination, even if you've decided to go somewhere else. Google maps doesn't appreciate you going off your programmed path, and nor does your brain.

Which is why when starting new patterns of behavior, it isn't easy and it's all too simple to fail and slide back to old patterns. Which is why I want to introduce you to an important theory called the Cycle of Change.

In my psychotherapy practice I use this in nearly all initial interactions with clients because I think it helps to give a sense of the journey while normalizing the ups-and-downs of change. Media skews what life is like for most people. If you watch TV adverts long enough, you'll think all it takes for life to become healthier is to swallow a pill or a chocolate shake. And if you do these simple tasks, you'll lose fifty pounds and reduce your blood sugar to normal levels. But that isn't the case.

Significant lifestyle changes take time, and consistent choices. Your journey will have many slips, trips and falls along the way to healthy blood. But that's normal because a slip-up now and then doesn't mean you're doing anything wrong.

Change is rarely a linear route, and for most us, it looks more like a crazy, shaky line with lots of peaks and troughs. And if you are one of those individuals who has multiple ups-and-downs while you're working on cleansing your blood, then I want to tell you that's how real change is and it's okay.

Here's a what a healthy change cycle looks like (adapted from the work by Prochaska and DiClemente[86]).

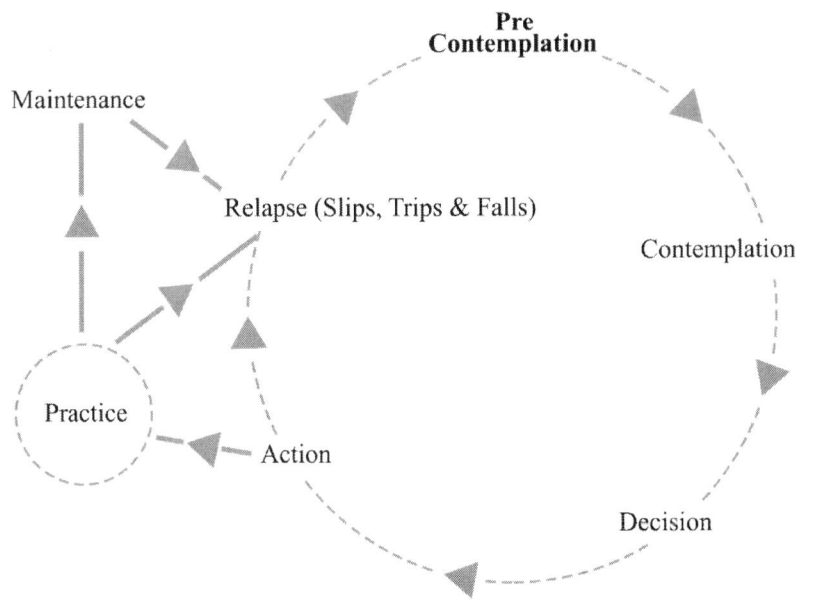

Pre-Contemplation

When you begin in this stage, you aren't thinking about change. In fact, the thought of change hasn't even entered your mind. This is the state you might have been before your doctor told you about your condition. Here, you are unaware of the change you are about to embark upon.

Contemplation

Here you have a seed of an idea about what you need to do to transform your condition to healthy. The thing about the contemplation stage is that you might be in it for seconds or even years. Sometimes you get that light-bulb moment and know what to do immediately, other times you sit with the what your next step might be. There really isn't a defined time-frame before you move to the next stage.

Decision

This part naturally follows the contemplation stage because we've thought about the problem and we decide to do something.

The decision phase still isn't quite the pivotal point of change. A decision to change is just that until we act. Just because you decide to change, it doesn't mean you'll automatically move forward into that space. Often when we don't act on that decision to change, we fall back into contemplation. Doubt and questions about the outcome can infuse our thinking again.

It is possible for someone to bounce between decision and contemplation over and over, not moving forward to action (although, taking no action is still action, but not forward-moving). This bouncing back and forth can continue for days, months or years and is usually because of fear or anxiety to change something.

If this is you, that's okay because sometimes we need to feel utterly stuck and frustrated with our lack of action before we finally push through our self-imposed roadblocks.

Action

Once the decision to move forward is firm we proceed to the action phase. What this means is you're now taking the necessary practical steps to start your change, and as the old proverb from Lao-tzu reminds us, 'A journey of a thousand miles begins with a single step'. This is what action is about. It's about taking the necessary step towards practicing your new behaviors. So, for somebody with your condition, taking action might be getting more sleep, or removing processed sugar from your diet.

Each phase in the cycle will be empowering, with the action phase having the most energy attached to it.

Practice

I've included this phase because I think after we've decided to do something, and we act on that decision, we need to practice our new action to become comfortable with it. Practice means we experiment with what we've changed, and we see what works for us and what doesn't. While practicing a new behavior we're becoming more comfortable with the changes we're making. We're getting feedback on what is and isn't working for us. Based on this feedback, we can adjust our behaviors accordingly to maintain a healthy, sustainable direction. I see this practice stage as an essential precursor to moving into the longer-term maintenance phase, which is the ongoing version of practice.

Remember, for all these cycles, once you step into one stage it doesn't mean you will be in it for hours or days at a time. In fact, you may practice your new behavior only once before you cycle through to relapse because something with the new behavior didn't stick. If that happens that's fine and part of the process.

You may even find you can practice your new behavior for several days or weeks extremely well before something happens and you cycle through to relapse. In time you will move to the maintenance stage.

Relapse

Relapse is often too strong a word, which is why I like to break it down into slips, trips, and falls. I'll cover that in a moment.

What relapse represents is sinking back into old behaviors for a considerable amount of time. Generally, if somebody is engaging in unhealthy old behaviors for a few months, I'd call that relapse. Usually after three or four months, you really need to start the change process from the beginning. However, that's not always a bad thing. Relapse can be a valuable experience because we do learn something on the way through the cycle. On reflection, we can determine why we relapsed. We may find our plan wasn't robust enough or we became complacent, letting ourselves slips a little more than was helpful. This awareness is invaluable to the long-term success of behavior change.

If you find you pass through the relapse stage a few times, then that's fine. With each cycle you'll learn what that relapse means to you and what you can do to avoid it next time.

Slips, Trips, and Falls

Because I see relapse as longer-term experience, I like to look at the concept of relapse as a series of steps on a spectrum. At one end of this spectrum you'll have what I call slips, and at the other end you'll have a full relapse. In between these two polarities there are a variety of trips and falls evenly spaced out.

I tell my clients that not every indiscretion or deviation from their program is a relapse. Relapse is more about completely ignoring your program and not doing anything to get back on track for a long period of time. A full relapse is typically followed by falling back into established, unhealthy patterns. Maybe not watching what they eat, staying up late or draining a six-pack with breakfast. A slip might be something like eating a candy bar every day for a few days before doing something to get back on plan.

Alternatively, a trip might be having a house guest for a week and making poor food choices for that duration. While a fall might be deviating from your program for a month, but you still get back on track before you let everything go too far.

The analogy I can offer for slips, trips, and falls is to imagine you're walking down an icy sidewalk. As you walk, you slip. Now a slip will make you momentarily lose your balance, but you can keep walking, maybe with slightly more caution. Now, imagine you are walking down the same sidewalk, but this time you catch your toe on uneven pavement and you trip forward. Again, this might be more forceful than the slip, but you stay on your feet and you cautiously keep walking.

And finally, you're still on the same icy sidewalk and this time you put your foot down and it slides in front of you and before you know it, you've tumbled onto your back. This is most definitely a fall and can cause damage and embarrassment. It might take more time to pick yourself up, but when you do, you will be really, really, cautious.

As you can see, slips, trips, and falls happen, even if we're being careful and doing all we can to maintain our equilibrium. It's the same with reversing your condition. I guarantee you'll slip, trip, and fall, but I hope you don't give up when these setbacks happen. If your health means something to you, then you get back on plan as soon as you can because the changes you are working on can save your life.

Maintenance

This is the off-ramp to the cycle of change. Maintenance is using new behaviors long enough for them to develop into your natural way of being.

Take learning to drive as an example. When you progress to the maintenance stage of driving, you're at the point of driving without having to think about it. You're not thinking about looking in your mirror, or how and when to stop or what the roadside signs mean. Everything is automatic.

Now, being in maintenance doesn't mean you won't slip, trip, fall or relapse, but if you do, you'll typically know enough to go back into maintenance almost immediately. If we take our driving analogy further; one day you might have an accident, you reverse into a parked car. This might be your first accident. So, what transpires next time you're reversing in a parking lot? You pay more attention when you back out. Maybe you take extra seconds to look behind you, and you do this because you learned a lesson from relapsing.

Although relapse is a pain in the backside and at moments can seem like you failed, it isn't failure if you take a moment to reflect. Learn what relapse has taught you and tell yourself you've relapsed because you had a lesson to learn about being more attentive to yourself and what keeps you healthy.

Building Your Team

Getting healthy and cleansing your blood will not only affect you, but those closest to you. And because of this, I think it helps to get friends and family involved in your journey because they can be supportive and keep you accountable. If you have a significant other, tell them immediately. Explain what you are embarking on and get them behind your plan. It also will help to have them read this book too.

I also recommend getting as many friends as possible on your team. If you have friends who you socialize with, then tell them your plan. If your friends know you're avoiding pizza, then good friends won't suggest going to a pizza parlor for a meal. Our friends are a good source of motivation on those days we don't feel like being healthy. A text or call can help bolster our defenses against the onslaught of temptation. It's difficult to make lifestyle choices, so allies are important.

You might also want to post something on social media. Let people know what you are doing and keep them updated on your progress. This might seem like sharing too much information or a risky step if you rarely follow through with plans, but these types of public proclamations can keep you accountable. Especially if you're not great at doing that for yourself. It's amazing how much support you can get when people know you are trying to get healthy. This support can be motivating.

How to Tell People

If you're not someone who feels comfortable telling people personal information, I get it. But I want to help you understand your change process. When you are not comfortable talking about yourself, then it helps to talk about yourself. Don't like feeling vulnerable, then feeling vulnerable. Doing certain activities we don't like to do, is a good way of becoming emotionally stronger. Avoiding parts of ourselves we would rather not have will not empower us. Avoidance makes us hide parts of who we are and that leads to emotional weakness and insecurity. Being authentic doesn't always mean being strong and smart for we are all fallible humans. Accepting we are fallible is an important part of the change process.

To overcome any initial awkwardness about telling people about your plans, I suggest creating a script. And the more you get used to talking about your plan, the more you'll say it with confidence. Here's a few starters.

- *"I'm making changes to my life to get healthier. This is a big deal to me, and I would be grateful for your support. I don't expect you to do all the things I do, but with your help I'll know I'll be more successful."*
- *"I found out I have diabetes, and I could use your help in keeping me accountable. If you see me stressing out, just tell me to calm down and breathe."*
- *"I wanted to let you know I'm planning to get healthy and take care of myself a little better. I have a plan and I feel good about it."*

Your script doesn't have to be full of information, but a little goes a long way in getting a helpful team together.

Unsupportive Family Members

The sad fact about change is that it won't excite everyone. Just because you're changing your lifestyle it doesn't mean your significant other is ready to go on that journey with you. If we look back at the cycle of change, you're at least at the action stage because you are reading this book. Your partner might be in the pre-contemplation stage because they're not even considering any lifestyle changes.

They might feel threatened by your change and this can lead to disagreements and even sabotaging behavior on their part. This behavior can be true if your significant other also has an unhealthy lifestyle. What happens is your desire to change, highlights parts of themselves that they aren't happy with, and might want to avoid. Maybe they need to lose weight, or quit smoking, or exercise more. They might feel your change process shines a light on them, and that might not be something they want to look at.

In these cases, the conflict in the beginning might seem difficult. However, in time, when your significant other or family member takes time to think about things, they move through the cycle of change and become supportive.

With a partner who is adamant they will not support you, then it's all on you to pull your socks up and make your own necessary changes. If you're used to your partner doing all the cooking, then it might be time for you to learn to cook for yourself. Responsibility for your own health is important and sets a good example. By showing them how serious you are, can change their attitude towards the process.

There isn't a quick fix to this challenge but stick to your plan. In my experience, they will eventually support you.

Unsupportive Friends

Just as family members can try to derail us, friends can too. Sometimes friends want to keep the relationship as it always was. If you have the friendships where you go out to eat, and drink together, they might see your cutting back or veering away from your typical choice, as threatening to the friendship. You might have that one friend who just doesn't know how to support you. They might say things like: "*Come on, it's only one beer, don't be so boring.*" It's like they can't accept you want to change and get healthy. And just as it was with the significant other, sometimes your change highlights parts of themselves that needs changing.

If these types of scenarios happen, then it's best to face it head-on and be clear with what you are trying to achieve by cleansing your blood. Having your scripts is always a good place to start. But there might be times when you might need extra help in shutting down a troublesome friend or a random person who doesn't accept your initial script.

I don't know why, but there is always that one friend or co-worker who always seems to think they know what's best for you. When faced with somebody like that, and you don't feel strong enough keeping your boundaries then I suggest adding a little white lie to your script. In my defense, I don't like lying and I don't advocate it, however, sometimes a slight massaging of the truth can help.

How to combat pushy people:

"I'd love to have that pizza with you, but my doctor is concerned about my blood work and I need to make changes. I'm following her plan to get healthy. If you want to have a pizza, I'll go with you. I just won't eat any."

And for the know-it-all:

"I appreciate your concern, and you have good ideas, but my doctor and I are working on a plan which for now, I'm sticking to."

The reason for invoking your doctors name is that most people won't question something that is a doctor's suggestion. When they hear a higher authority is guiding you, they'll accept it. They may not like it, and they may question your doctor's judgment, but they'll stop pushing because you can always invoke, 'doctor's orders,' anytime you get push-back.

Creating A Benefits List

Of all the tasks in this book, the benefits list is the most important. If you do nothing else, I encourage you to do this. The reason for creating a benefits list is so you have something you can refer to when things get challenging or boring, because they inevitably will. It's just a natural part of the process. When those moments of waning motivation happen, accessing your original motivation will give you enough energy to get you over the proverbial hump.

A good benefits list needs emotional investment to be powerful. Too often when people want to change something, they focus on the goal rather than the benefits. I've heard people set goals of: *"I want to lose weight,"* or *"I want to get healthy"* or *"I don't want to be diabetic anymore."* These are fine goals, but they are not benefits, and they don't have the same power to help you change.

The difference between benefits and a goal is that a goal is something you aim to achieve but is less specific than a benefit. A benefit is something tangible you can explain and almost feel physically when you think about it. Goals and benefits work together, but we know what your goal is if you're reading this book. We know you want to reverse your blood condition, but what isn't clear is what will you gain from reaching that goal.

Let me show you how to make your benefits specific, with an example conversation with a client as he creates his own list.

Benefits Conversation with JD

DC: JD, what personal benefits do you want to gain regarding being on this program?

JD: I guess I don't want to be diabetic anymore.

DC: That would be great but that isn't a benefit, it's more of a negative-focused goal which will not help you much on those days where you feel less motivated or bored. And what I mean by a negative-focused goal is that you start the premise of change with what you don't want, rather than what would be better for you when you are healthier. That goal is fine for things like I want a new car, or I want a new job but when we are talking about behavior change, we need a stronger motivation that resonates within our core. So, we want to look at what you'll gain from all the work you'll put into being healthy. How about we re-frame this goal into a benefit? Let me ask you a few questions and we'll see if we can flesh it out a little.

JD: Sounds good.

DC: Okay, so you don't want to be diabetic. Now if you weren't diabetic, what benefit would you gain from not being diabetic?

JD: Well, I guess I wouldn't take medication every day which often makes me feel nauseous. I'd be more energetic, and I wouldn't have the crappy fatigue I have most of the time. Plus, I might even live longer.

DC: They all seem preferable to being diabetic. What you've said all sounds like it's linked with you feeling better physically?

JD: Yeah, that is a goal. I'm 50 but most days I feel like I'm 90.

DC: Cool. So, let's imagine you're not taking medication anymore, and you're feeling better. What would be different in your life? What would be the upsides, the benefits, of feeling better?

JD: Oh, so many things. I have two grandchildren who I adore, and I'd love to have more energy to play with them; to be around them and watch them grow-up. I'd also have more energy to get back to hiking the hills and forests near our house with my wife and dog. I think being able to get out and be more active would be fun. Oh, and I'd also love to go on a long cruise with my wife as it's something we've been talking about for years. I think that would be fantastic. To go away and not have to worry about my medication or being sick or tired when I'm away.

DC: Wow, that sounds great. I think it's fair to say there are many good things to look forward to when you're healthier. And when you think of having the energy to play with your grandchildren, walking the hills and forests with your wife and going on a long cruise, how do you feel?

JD: Excited. Ready to go.

DC: Excellent. So, would it be better to focus on the negative-focused goal of 'I don't want to be diabetic anymore', or would it be better to focus on the benefit of 'I'll have more energy to play with my grandchildren and watch them grow, go walking in the hills and forests with my wife and dog, and to go on a cruise and see the world without the worry of being sick'?

JD: Oh, the last ones for sure. Every time I think of those benefits, I do feel as if I have a great future.

DC: Fantastic. Here we have three positive and realistic benefits for the price of one negative-focused goal. What we need to do now is to write these down. I want you to look at these at least once a week. And when you look at your benefits list, I'd like you to close your eyes and feel how good it would be to do all those things, okay?

JD: Absolutely.

> **I want to be well so...**
> I'll have more energy to play with my grandchildren and watch them grow.
>
> I'll also be there when they are old enough to get married in 20 years or so.
>
> **I want to be well so...**
> I'll have more energy to walk with my wife and dog over the forest and hills. And go hiking with friends in the summer.
>
> **I want to be well so...**
> I'll have the energy to go on that long cruise with my wife and see some amazing places, while spending time with the love of my life.

As you can see from this quick exchange with JD, we took his simple, yet not inspiring goal and, in a few seconds, brought to life the benefits he would gain by cleansing his blood. What I'd like you to do now is to take a moment to write at least three benefits of your own, just like JD.

You might start with the same train of thought JD had with: **I don't want to be...** then ask yourself: *"What would be different in my life if I didn't have my condition? What benefits would I gain from this?"*

Keep asking yourself that question until you have three benefits that fire you up. Because for these benefits to have power, they need to hit you in your heart. You need to see yourself living these benefits and know why you're doing this program because these benefits will help you have the strength of will and consistency to face any challenge that comes along.

I encourage you dig deep and spend a good amount of time on this, because you might surprise yourself with what you want for yourself, and your life. There's something more permanent when we write something down long-hand. It's like making it real in our brain. Once you've written your benefits, stick your sheet somewhere that you'll see it every day. That reminder is powerful in the long-run. You might even want to set a reminder on your phone or computer to pop up once a week as another visual aide-mémoire.

Potential Fears and Challenges

Now you have three benefits (and maybe more), the next step of our action plan is to address any fears you might have about potential obstacles to reversing your condition.

Let's go back to JD and look at how he created his list.

DC: Right, we have our benefits list, and now I want to look at fears and concerns. I may sound like the Grinch here, but I want to make sure that if something does come along which challenges you, you'll know how to deal with it. Okay?
JD: Sure, sounds good.
DC: Great, so let's take your first benefit as a starting point because I think all your other benefits will probably be related to the fears and concerns you might have about the first one. Your first benefit was, 'I'll have more energy to play with my grandchildren and watch them grow and be there when they get married in 20 years'. Again, a fantastic benefit, but let me ask you this: what potential fears or concerns do you have about not attaining this benefit of having the energy to play with your grandchildren or live to see them get married?
JD: Um, well, I guess I worry that I won't stick to my plan, and by not doing that I'll fail. Yeah, I guess I am concerned that I'll fail my wife and grandchildren.
DC: Anything else you're fearful of?
JD: I guess I'm fearful that I'll give in and not finished the program because I've done that before. I've started so many diets and done well but I soon get bored and start snacking on chips and ice cream

again, and I know I can't do that if I want to experience those good things with my family.

DC: Okay. Let me outline that again so we know what we're dealing with. You're afraid of letting your wife and grandchildren down if you get bored and start snacking again which typically leads to you falling off the wagon and ditching your diet. You're also afraid of this happening because it's happened before. Is that right?

JD: Absolutely.

DC: Right, so let's break this down a little more. Take your piece of paper and draw two columns. The first column is for Potential Fears/Concerns and the second column is How They Can Be Handled. In the first column, I want you to write down, 'Fear of failing and slipping back into old habits'. Okay?

JD: Okay, done.

DC: So how are you going to deal with your fear of failing and slipping back?

JD: Um, not fail?

DC: Wouldn't that be easy. Let me put it this way, what's so bad about failing?

JD: It's terrible. I hate failing and I'd hate for my family to be disappointed in me.

DC: Would they be?

JD: No. Well, maybe a little.

DC: Let's say you do disappoint them, that's not the end of the world is it?

JD: Not really. But it's not good.

DC: Not good but definitely not terrible?

JD: No, not terrible.

DC: So how are you going to deal with disappointing them?

JD: Well, typically I'd probably try and ignore it, but I know me, I start eating crap when I feel guilty or sad.

DC: So disappointing people leads you to punish yourself by eating badly.

JD: Yes.

DC: And if you eat badly, what happens to you?

JD: I feel worse, my diabetes gets worse and then I just feel more ashamed.

DC: So, we could say your strategy for dealing with failure and disappointing people is to make yourself sicker, which means you're less likely to have the energy to play with your grandchildren, walk the dog and go on a cruise, which will lead to more guilt and disappointment.

JD: Ah, yeah. I get what you're saying.

DC: Alright. Let's assume you do fall off the wagon a bit and eat badly for a day or two, and you do disappoint your family, what are you going to do to overcome this behavior and challenge your typical reaction?

JD: If I eat badly for a few days, then I need to just stop, accept that I'm not going to be perfect, accept that my behavior is disappointing and get back on track with my plan because that is best for me and my family in the long-run.

DC: And what about your feelings of failure.

JD: I guess I haven't really failed if I get back on track.

DC: Very true. So, we can look at it this way; I'm concerned that I'll slip up and eat badly but if I do it's not the end of the world, just disappointing. However, I'll remind myself why I want to get well, and the benefits of getting well. I'll make sure I take steps to start following my plan again because slipping up now and then isn't failing, it's just a blip in the process.

JD: Yes, I can do that.

DC: Write those down and anything else you can think of.

> **Potential Fears & Concerns:**
> Fear of failing and slipping back into old habits.
>
> **How Can They Be Handled?**
> Remind myself it's not the end of the world to fail, even if it is disappointing.
>
> If I do slip up, I'll remind myself to review my Benefits List and remember why I want to be well. I'll then start doing what I need to get healthier.
>
> ---
>
> **Potential Fears & Concerns:**
> Feeling guilty and disappointing my family for not sticking to my plan.
>
> **How Can They Be Handled?**
> Accept that I may not always be perfect, and if I do feel guilty, understand that I do tend to eat badly which makes my problem worse.
>
> Tell myself that the old ways don't work for me and I can rectify that by getting back on plan ASAP!

As you can see from this exchange, I wanted to help JD understand that things don't always go to plan. We do screw up and slip – and that's okay as long as we take steps to rectify what we know is unhealthy behavior. It's one thing to slip up and throw in the towel, it's another to slip up and get back on track. Remember, slips, trips and falls are all part of a health Cycle of Change.

What I'd like you to do is the same thing as JD. I'd like you to start thinking about all the things you're concerned about regarding getting well. You might think you don't have any concerns, and that's okay, just spend a little bit of time reflecting on previous experiences when you've tried to change something in your life and ask questions like what you did that helped, and what behaviors you did when things went awry.

If you want a Potential Fears & Concerns worksheet, you can print a copy from my website drewcoster.com/worksheets

Potential Obstacles

This is the final part of our plan. In this section, I want to look at those obstacles and roadblocks that might arise over the coming months while you're still working on getting into healthy routines. These can be things like traveling, business dinners, or boredom. Later, I'll talk about some of these usual challenges and add some tips on how to manage them but for now, I'd like to focus on what your potential obstacles are and how you plan to deal with them.

For this, we're going back to my conversation with JD.

DC: Right, the last hurdle. I'd like us to think about potential obstacles you might face over the coming weeks and months. I'd then like us to think about how you can overcome these obstacles and stay on track.
JD: Sure.
DC: So, thinking about the next month or two, do you have anything going on that might be a potential obstacle?
JD: Oh yeah, loads.
DC: Such as?
JD: In two weeks my wife and I are going to her mother's for a week and she fries everything. I don't want to be rude and not have what she makes us, so I know from experience that I usually eat whatever she makes.
DC: Okay. Anything else?
JD: I guess I have a couple of working lunches in the next few weeks, but I know I can manage those. Oh, we do have a few birthdays every month in my office which means we tend to have a lot of cake sitting around, which I find hard for me to turn down.

DC: Well, that'll get us started. On your sheet of paper, I'd like you to draw another box with two columns. The first column is Potential Obstacles and the second is How I'll Overcome Them. When you've done that, in the Obstacles column write down what you told me; eating at my mother-in-law's; cake in the office (for the purpose of time, we'll just deal with the cake issue).

JD: Okay.

DC: Now, let's take the cake obstacle. How do you think you'll overcome that one?

JD: I just won't have any.

DC: Really?

JD: Yeah... well, I don't know. This kind of ties in with my fear of failing.

DC: One thing I'd like you to remember is that this is a lifestyle change, not a trip to purgatory. What I mean by that is whenever we tell ourselves that we absolutely can't have something, or we try to stick rigidly to our self-made rules, we're more likely to slip and fall rather than if we let ourselves enjoy a little of what we want now and then. Does that make sense?

JD: Yeah it does. I often do that to myself. I put myself in a black and white situation and when I don't follow my rules, I then chastise myself for failing, and that makes things worse.

DC: Right, exactly. Imagine there's cake in your office and you tell yourself that you absolutely can't have any, how do you think you'll feel about that?

JD: I guess I'd be afraid of the cake. Afraid that I'd give in and have some. And if I do that, I know I'll just have more and more because at that point I'm back to eating my guilt over failing.

DC: Good. Now imagine you said to yourself, I can have a little cake if I want because it's not the end of the world if I do.

JD: I'd probably feel more relaxed about it. But then that might be my excuse to eat a lot.

DC: And if you do eat a lot?

JD: Ah, I'm back to my failure loop.

DC: Indeed. Look, the best way to tackle this type of obstacle is to accept that you can have some cake if you choose. I don't want you to be afraid of food, because when you become afraid of food, that food has control over you; and that's just silly. You give yourself permission to have some or not, and whichever you choose is your responsibility, and that choice puts you in control.

JD: I can see that.

DC: Right, so imagine you have cake in your office every day for a month. How are you going to overcome that?

JD: When I think of having some cake or not, I feel a lot more relaxed about it. Actually, the idea of having a lot of cake is a bit of a turn off now that I know what it does to me. I don't think I'd like any.

DC: And if you do want some?

JD: Then I'll have a bit. No big deal.

DC: Go ahead and write that down.

Potential Obstacles I Might Face:
Cake in the office!!

How I'll Overcome Them?
I'll try and avoid it as much as I can, but if I find I want a piece then I will only have a bite or two.

If I eat more than that, then I will remind myself how damaging sugar is for me and how this piece of cake is sabotaging all the benefits of getting well.

There you have it, our quick and easy benefits list with potential challenges. Doing this short exercise will give you a better understanding of how you 'work' when faced with challenges, and having strong, emotionally stirring benefits to refer to in the face of any challenges.

If you want a Potential Obstacles worksheet, you can print a copy from my website drewcoster.com/worksheets

Recognize Emotional Eating

Emotional eating tends to happen as a result of experiencing negative emotions. The triggers for emotional eating tend to come from boredom, sadness, and loneliness. Food is used as a mood pick-me-up and is a way to sabotage your plan to be healthy. Emotional eating is also sometimes called stress eating as it is a way to deflect how we feel into food.

If you've ever sat in front of the TV and mindlessly thrown popcorn into your mouth after a hard day at work, then you'll understand what emotional eating is. If you're sitting at home alone and you grab a pint of ice cream and slowly work your way through it without realizing you've finished it, you are emotional eating. It doesn't matter what your trigger is, it's how emotional eating can impact your blood and your health.

To get a sense if you are an emotional eater, answer these questions.

1. Do you eat a specific type of food when you are sad, bored, stress or lonely?
2. Do you eat more than would be considered a single serving?
3. Do you often find you've finished the tub or packet of food without realizing you've eaten so much?
4. Do you still want more after you've finished?
5. Does food feel like a comfort when you're down?
6. Do you feel powerless around food when you are sad, bored, stress or lonely?

If you answered yes to all or nearly all, then I think it's safe to say you are an emotional eater. The good news is that we can learn to recognize when we are emotional eating and take appropriate steps to stop or at least reduce the potential damage overeating has on your blood.

The first thing to do is not give yourself a hard time if you are an emotional eater. Emotional eating for many has filled a void. A way for them to feel safe and soothed in the face of emotional adversity. Not everyone is taught how to deal with their emotions and food, for many, is an easy friend in times of stress.

Food is typically used as a way to stuff down feelings or to fill a void. Have you ever passed a food shop and smelt or seen something and immediately thought that would be great to eat? What you'll also notice is how quickly a feeling of happiness comes over you. I know when I walk past a pizza store, I can feel myself smile when I look at the slices. It's not that I'm hungry, but the idea of eating pizza lifts my mood and makes me happy. This is the power of emotional eating.

The Difference Between Physical Hunger & Emotional Eating

There is a very simple self-assessment you can do to quickly know if you are truly physically hungry because your ghrelin hormone has kicked in, or if you want to eat because of an emotional trigger.

Physical Hunger

- You will feel the desire for food come from your stomach and not your head.
- Physical hunger comes on slowly. Often with some rumbling in your stomach to remind you to eat.
- Physical hunger isn't about a specific food.
- When you are physically hungry you aren't as choosy and will eat anything.

- You'll feel physically satisfied after eating and you stop thinking about food.

Emotional Hunger

- Typically comes from your head.
- The feeling you suddenly get will be of happiness or excitement.
- It is a sudden and overwhelming desire for a specific food.
- You'll then fixate on this food until you get it.
- You won't necessarily feel full after eating.
- You might also feel shame or guilt or regret after eating.

Steps to Understanding Emotional Eating

Step One:

To understand your own emotional eating, first you'll need to identify which unhealthy negative emotion you are feeling and then we can pair the associated food you eat with that emotion. For example, when you are stressed you might choose pizza. When sad, chocolate cookies. Because these emotions and foods are often different, you'll probably want to go through this exercise for each unhealthy negative emotion you recognize you emotionally eat to.

Step Two:

Next, we want to know which food you choose when this unhealthy negative emotion kicks in. Typical emotions that trigger food cravings are sad, bored, stress or lonely but you may have something different. It might help to make a list and compare the food you choose to the emotion you feel.

Step Three:

Try and understand how you feel eating this emotional food. Often you can do this with your imagination. Close your eyes and imagine eating the food you choose when you're sad. Pay attention to how your brain lights up and how instantly happy you feel. You might feel your mouth turning into a smile. Even just doing this shows the power of emotional eating.

Step Four:

Now we know the negative emotion you feel, the food you choose to soothe yourself, and the alternative positive emotion this new food summons. The next step is to understand if there is a positive memory invoked when you eat your emotionally charged food. The reason for this is because we want to understand how your brain is using a happy past experience to overwrite what negative feeling you currently have. This will ultimately inform you on what healthy alternative action you can take to counter your negative emotion, that doesn't include reaching for a pint of Phish Food.

Step Five:

Now you understand your emotion, your emotional eating pattern and what positive emotion your brain is making you feel to counter the negative one, you'll want to figure out what you can do instead of eating to feel better. For example, if you are feeling bored, then engage in an activity you enjoy. Maybe exercise or go for a walk. If you're feeling sad, write your feelings down or talk to a friend. Something that helps get your thoughts and feelings out. Doing something is better than doing nothing while eating to replace your negative unhealthy emotion.

Doing something may not solve the solution to your unhealthy emotions in the long-term, but neither will be eating a pepperoni pizza and chugging a bottle of wine. Once you can recognize your sabotaging habits, as well meaning as these habits are, the easier it will be for you to choose healthy alternative that will help sustain lifestyle change and balance your Five Pillars.

My Example:

- When I feel lonely, I want to eat ice cream.
- When I think of eating ice cream, I feel happy.
- Behind this emotional food is a memory of being about 9 years old and sitting around the dining room table with my family. I have a happy feeling in my chest as I squirt chocolate sauce all over my ice cream.
- To counter this loneliness, it would be healthier for me to call a friend. Even a brief conversation will give me a sense of connection.

This memory is my emotional eating anchor, and it's a way for my brain to quickly counter any negative emotions I feel. Even though I don't think of the memory when I eat ice cream, the association is strong enough that I instantly feel happy when I eat it because in my brain my loneliness has been replaced by a memory of being with family. Eating ice cream is often enough to reduce my loneliness for a short time, but this isn't a long-term solution, which is why you need to explore alternative which are more sustainable and fulfilling.

Also, if any of these emotionally charged foods are on the NO list later in the book, then you know these foods will be even more of a challenge to work around because of the carb or sugar content making your brain feel happy. But don't worry, emotional eating is very common, but you can get to grips with this. Learning how and why you do things which may ordinarily be out of your awareness will help you overcome emotional eating. These emotionally charged foods are also Trigger Foods, which we'll look at next.

> **Unhealthy Negative Emotion Experiencing?**
> Loneliness.
>
> **Emotionally Charged Food Choice?**
> Ice cream.
>
> **Positive Feeling From Emotional Eating?**
> I feel happy.
> Ice cream feels like a good friend who's always there.
>
> **Memory Evoked?**
> Eating dinner with my whole family as a child, and the excitement of having a bowl of ice cream as a Sunday treat.
>
> **Alternative Healthy Action?**
> Call a friend or family member to feel connected.

If you want an Emotionally Charged Foods worksheet, you can print a copy from my website drewcoster.com/worksheets

Managing Trigger Foods

Like Emotional Eating, Trigger Foods are the type of food we eat that 'trigger' us to eat more than is healthy portion. Emotional eating and trigger foods sometimes share the same food choices, but they often have different functions. Where emotional eating is about filling a void and self-soothing, trigger foods tend to be more about loss of control and overeating. For some people their trigger is sweet foods like chocolate, for others savory crackers, or crunchy chips. It doesn't really matter what food it is, there's something about it that will trigger you to keep eating even when you've had enough.

The reason trigger food is a problem is because, whatever your food choice, it's going to propel your brain into its happy, high-as-a-kite place. The crux of the matter is trigger foods tend to be quick carbs and sugar, and these are somewhat addictive substances.[2,5,4,80]

What makes sugar such an addictive type of food, is that it raises our dopamine levels, which creates a dopamine reward feedback loop. What this means is if you eat something that's pleasurable (not necessarily sugar), your brain will want it again and again. And what this feedback loop shows is that our brain isn't passive in our food choices. On the contrary, the brain will 'like' and 'want' certain foods over others, putting a preference on foods which are sweet.[80,81,82]

This reward loop will make choosing food which don't have a high sugar content (or high sugar from carbohydrates) difficult because our desire for that sweetness will make other foods seem bland and unappealing. Faced with a chocolate cookie or a stick of celery, which do you chose? You may look at the choices, and your thinking brain may consider the celery as the rational, healthier option. However, your sweet-addicted, hedonistic brain will overrule your choice and make you go for the chocolate, even if you know that it's a poor decision.

Dopamine Reward Loop

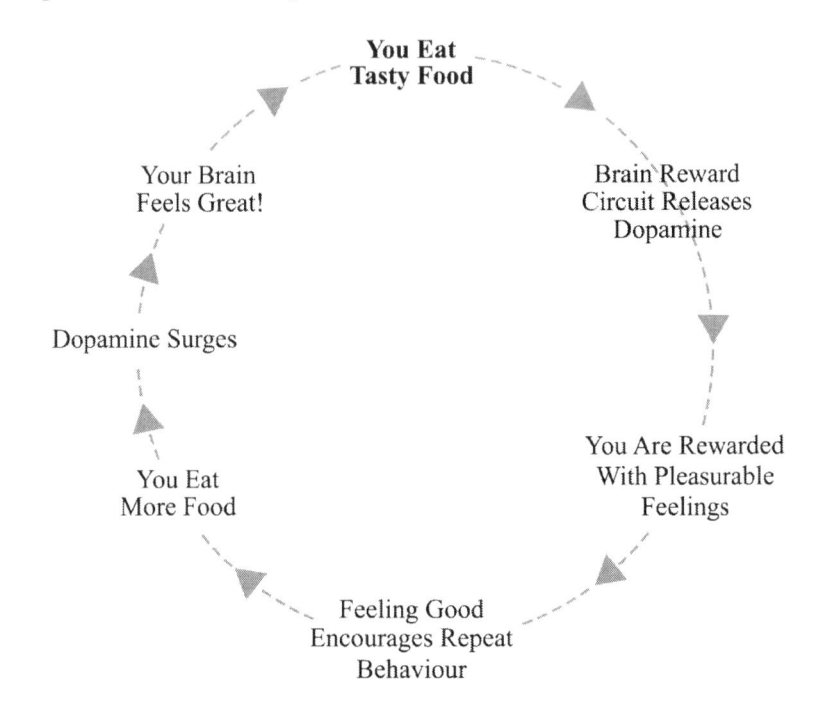

```
                    You Eat
                   Tasty Food

   Your Brain                      Brain Reward
   Feels Great!                    Circuit Releases
                                   Dopamine


  Dopamine Surges

                                   You Are Rewarded
   You Eat                         With Pleasurable
   More Food                       Feelings


                  Feeling Good
                Encourages Repeat
                    Behaviour
```

The annoying thing about trigger foods and the reward loop is how much of a hold it has over us. It's the type of food we'll see in a TV advert and start craving it as soon as we see the images. Or you might be in a restaurant, and even though you planned to eat a balanced meal, you end up ordering something that looks great and ticks all your trigger food boxes, even if you know your blood sugar is going to suffer. Because of this link to our brain, trigger foods can be so destructive and such a hard habit to break.

One of my trigger foods is pizza. I often tell myself: "*Just one slice will be a nice treat.*" But that one slice turns into eating the whole large pizza. More like six to eight slices. After eating I know I made a mistake in my choice because I feel lousy – physically, emotionally and cognitively. But does that stop me ordering it again, even if I don't really want it? Nope. As soon as someone suggests we get pizza, I'm all in. Just saying the word pizza means I'm triggered. I can't stop. The dopamine reward loop in my brain means the more I eat, the more pleasure I feel and the more I want. I only really stop once it is all gone, otherwise I would keep going.

It took me a long time to be able to look at a pizza and not have it. Don't get me wrong, I do have some now and then, and I still love it, until I've finished and then I regret my decision. I'm also better drive past a pizza place without getting excited, but I do sometimes have to talk my triggered brain out of stopping. This is partially why it is hard for drug and alcohol abusers to stay clean and sober.

What we don't want to do is be afraid of food, even if it triggers us. Because once we are afraid, then that food will have total control over us and that really doesn't make sense. I also know avoiding any type of food can lead to cravings and resentment in the long run, so we need to find some middle ground when it comes to Trigger Foods.

In the beginning of your journey to cleanse your blood, I do recommend you avoid buying or trying any and all of your trigger foods for at least two to three months. Because abstaining from something we enjoy can trigger cravings, you might want to let your brain know this abstinence is only temporary. This might sound odd, but often to overcome habits, especially trigger food habits, we need to first negotiate with our brain. The best way to do this is to articulate out loud something like this: "*I know I really enjoy XYZ food, and I also know this food isn't good for me. So, for now, I'm going skip buying it for three months. I'm doing this to break my habit from this food. If after three months I feel I can have a taste here and there, I will, and if I don't want it ever again, that's fine too.*"

What we're doing by saying this out loud is making sure our brain hears us. As weird as that sounds, when we articulate things out loud, they have far more power than when we think them. We're telling our frontal cortex, the bit that experiences the dopamine reward, that we are just taking a 'vacation' from our favorite foods and it's not going to be forever. In many ways, talking to our brain is like talking to a needy child. Explain everything in an adult voice and you'll be surprised how much you brain accepts your decision. But think about changing something, and your brain will often out vote you with sneaky suggestions.

By taking a break from eating trigger foods, you are also giving your body and mind a chance to lose interest in that food. Typically, after two or three months the desire to eat a certain trigger food diminishes to the point it doesn't interest you anymore. Even having a gap from a trigger food can mean when we do eat it again, it might not taste the same as you remember. This is often because our taste bud cells naturally expire after two weeks and are replaced with new cells. These new cells will taste food differently if you haven't had it for a while. The new taste buds will also be okay with less sweet food like salad if you've removed a lot of sweet stuff from your diet. You might be surprised at how amazing different foods are when we refrain from the sweet stuff for a while.

Identifying Trigger Foods

Once you get past that two or three-month mark without a trigger food, you'll either feel confident that you don't need or want it anymore; or you might be in the position that you'd like to have it as a treat now and then. When we do get to the point of testing ourselves, we need to be prepared, so let's try another exercise.

First, make a list of all your trigger foods. These may also be the same as your emotionally eating foods.

> **Trigger Foods:**
>
> Ice cream
>
> Chocolate, especially Lindor or Swiss chocolate
>
> Bread, especially toast
>
> Pizza
>
> Cakes, cookies, biscuits
>
> Chocolate muffins
>
> Cereals, especially Cocoa Puffs
>
> Any sugary food!

The only way we can test your control over trigger foods is to eat some. You might feel a little apprehensive at this idea, knowing how quickly things can get out of control, but don't worry. The first couple of times you try this exercise you might slip and have more than you planned but you won't go back to square one. In the event that this goes really badly, then you might have to take a few steps back and refrain from trigger food again for a few more weeks. But with practice and understanding how these foods impact you, you are in a terrific place to see just how damaging these food choices can be.

The way to approach understanding your trigger foods is to ask yourself these questions:

Before Eating Trigger Foods

1. What thoughts are going through your mind before you eat this Trigger Food?
2. What sensation are you feeling in your body?
3. What's going on in your brain and what's happening in your stomach?

Now you have these answers it's time to eat a small amount. If your trigger food is chocolate, then just have a piece or two. If it's ice cream, then one large tablespoon. Keep whatever your food choice is to a very manageable portion. Don't be scared at this point, instead allow yourself to be curious. Imagine this is research, and you're trying to find out what impact this food has on you, whether that's a positive or negative experience. Once you've eaten your trigger food, ask yourself these questions.

After Eating Trigger Foods

1. Were you able to stick to one piece of Trigger Food and put the rest away?
2. If so, what are you thinking and feeling now?
3. If you had more than one piece, what are you thinking and feeling now?
4. How do you think this experiment went?

If all went well, you'll have eaten a little of your trigger food and put the rest away. If you did, congratulations this is a big step and will help you approach trigger food with a different mindset in the future.

If you didn't do so well and ate more than you planned, don't worry, at least you know this is a strong trigger food for you. If things didn't go to plan, then don't put pressure on yourself. In time and with practice, you'll overcome this challenge too. In the meantime, go through these questions and reflect upon what your experience was.

Questions When Things Don't Go to Plan:

1. What was your sensory experience when you picked up and ate the Trigger Food (sight, smell, taste)?
2. What went through your mind after eating the first bite?
3. What went through your mind after you had eaten the second bite?

4. What went through your mind after eating all your Trigger Food?
5. What happened to make you stop eating the Trigger Food?
6. What was your physical experience after eating your Trigger Food?
7. What did you think about yourself once you had finished the Trigger Food?
8. Did you give yourself a tough time after? Did you call yourself names?

These questions will help you learn more about your thinking, behavior and emotions when it comes to food your brain really likes. In time, we want to get to the point where you're are at least more cognizant of what you are choosing to eat and the effect it has on you. I would encourage you to try this exercise again in about a month to see what's changed. Some changes to the food we eat takes a lot more time than others, and it might be that there are some foods you'll always struggle with. Pizza anyone?

I would be lying if I told you I had complete control over all my trigger foods because I don't. Most of the time, I'm totally fine, but there are those moments, usually over the holidays or when I'm overly tired, when I tend to lose control and have way more of my trigger foods than is good for me. However, progress not perfection. If I find I'm able to stop from going too far and take strides to minimize the damage I'm doing to myself, I feel pretty good about myself. And yes, this is also a tough thing to do. Sometimes I win, sometimes I lose, but that's life. Each time you lose the battle to trigger food, try and understand why. What was the trigger, is an important question?

One of the biggest lessons I hope you learn from understanding your trigger food is the impact they have on you physically, cognitively and emotionally. And if you've ever had the thought: *"Well, I've made a bad food choice and completely blown it. I might as well keep eating."* Then that thought isn't helpful and is more about self-sabotage than anything else. You're better off admitting what's happened and take strides to alter how you think about making a less than helpful choice. Maybe reframe your thinking like this: "*I've eaten way too many XYZ, but I can stop, and I will. I know this is tough for me, but I'm not going to make it worse by repeating an unhealthy behavior by keep going.*"

Just keep working away and learn to understand your trigger foods and how to manage them. In time, who knows, maybe you'll be able to ditch them for good.

Exception Eating

Although trigger foods can lead to overeating, it doesn't mean we have to give up these foods forever and not indulge ourselves once in a while. I often refer to having 'treat meals' or 'treat food' now and again because I think it's important to still enjoy some foods which might be in the NO list in the Nutrition section. However, there is still this big caveat - in moderation.

Eating treat foods are what I call Exception Eating, and this means foods which we know are not good for our blood but occasionally we make an exception to have them. There are two types of exception eating: *planned* and *unplanned*.

Planned Exception Eating

This is when you know you're going to a party or you're going out for dinner, and you plan to have a treat that you know isn't the best choice. It might be that you are planning to have some pizza or a dessert with your kids, or you plan to have champagne and cake at a friend's wedding.

These planned exceptions are okay now and then because you've made a choice to do this. And with that rational choice comes more control over what and how much you eat. These exceptions are also good for the brain, so it doesn't get bored from abstinence. If I know in advance that I have a treat meal to look forward to, then it makes it easier to avoid many other trigger foods throughout the week. This is what makes the 'treat exception' even more enjoyable because I can look forward to having it. I can even plan it and build up my anticipation for it, which makes it even more enjoyable.

These exceptions are something I encourage all my clients to indulge in now and then because I think it's reasonable to assume that you are human and as such, you're unlikely to follow this plan 100% without losing your mind. When you're planning exception eating, it can help to studying the restaurant menu a day or two beforehand and making sure you know what you're going to order before you get there.

By deciding upon your choice ahead of time, you don't need to look at the menu which will limit any temptation to waiver from your choice. Another thing can do the day after you have your exception meal, is keep as close to your healthy eating plan as possible. No deviation. This way you won't let that exception meal leak into the next day which it can do if you are not prepared.

Eating high carb food can make you crave more carbs the next day, which is why being more concerted to make healthy choices the next day is important. Which leads us to the other type of exception eating, unplanned exceptions.

Unplanned Exception Eating

This is when you go out (or you're maybe at home) and you start to eat food you know isn't on your plan and isn't good for your blood. Typically, this is when you go for your trigger food. I find fatigue can be a big factor for me, or if I've not eaten for several hours and I'm overly hungry. Which is why I never recommend going grocery shopping hungry because you'll always buy things you wouldn't if you didn't shop hungry.

This also goes for restaurants. Never go out hungry because it's way too easy to order everything on the menu that you know is bad for your blood. You will have less control over your choices when you're hungry.

Unplanned Exception Eating is the most destructive of the two because at least with a planned exception you know what you're having, and you have a modicum of control. With unplanned eating, it can be a free-for-all that can quickly become overwhelming. Plus, after we've finished our unplanned exception, we might start having negative thoughts and feelings about ourselves and our uncontrolled behavior.

These thoughts can then have a knock-on effect of triggering emotional eating. If I've felt disappointed in myself after an unplanned exception, then it's not fun to then beat myself up about it. It's always better to know that you're going to have a treat rather than just lose control, because as soon as you lose control, your brain takes over like the sugar junkie it is. Before you know it, you're stuck in that dopamine reward loop.

By now you understand what emotional eating is, and what your trigger foods are. Knowing this won't necessarily stop you from any unplanned exception eating but if you don't buy the foods which trigger you, then there is less chance of overeating on the bad stuff.

Do yourself a favor, and plan some exception throughout the month, your brain will thank you for it.

Self-Care Action Plan

It still astonishes me how many of my clients don't put time aside for things they enjoy throughout the week. They tend to do all they can to fill their week by focusing on other people's needs first. And while this is great in an altruistic sense, it's not entirely helpful if you want to be healthy. Self-Care is essential for good long-term health and wellbeing.

What do I mean by Self-Care? Simple really – you do something you enjoy that's just for you every day or at least a few times a week. Yes, I know, you don't have time, well this is the problem – time.

Time is precious and if you have young children who have multiple activities after school, then you know how little time you have rushing between activities. But I'm here to tell you, unless you carve out a little time for self-care, you're not doing yourself justice.

Typically, when I talk about a self-care action plan, I'm told two things: "*I don't have time to do more in the day*" and "*I don't want to be selfish*" My response is always the same, self-care is absolutely not the same as selfishness. In fact, it's the opposite. Selfishness is lacking any consideration about others and profiting by this. Self-Care is about making sure you are well and healthy so that you're more available to help others.

I understand it can be easy to get our sense of self-worth from doing for others. I spent a good deal of my life doing just that because giving feels good, but I challenge you to learn that an important part of self-care is to let others give to you. This may be a tough lesson, but it's an important one for personal growth. When we can do good things for ourselves, we are in a much better place to help others. Self-Care means we have a stronger, and most importantly, healthy foundation for giving and receiving.

One of the misconceptions of self-care is that you need to spend hours doing it to gain any benefit. As nice as that would be, most of us don't have that luxury. So how much time do you need for self-care? I think even 10 minutes a day is a good start if you really are pushed for time. But rather than trying to stuff more into your day, I always find it is a good exercise to see how you can do less in a day. That might sound crazy, but when we analyze a typical day, you might be surprised at how much time is spent on activities that could be changed, reduced or even delegated to somebody else.

Most people don't think about what they do in a day and how many hours are allocated to different tasks, but I find doing this helpful. The best way to incorporate Self-Care into your day is sometimes about being more efficient with what time you have available.

Below is an exercise I did with a client called Susan, a single mother with a twelve-year-old son. Susan was terrible at self-care and this had a knock-on effect to her health, leading to prediabetes.

Where Does the Time Go?

In this exercise we want to figure out what a typical day looks like and then adjust to make room for self-care. Remember, self-care doesn't mean hours a day. The idea is to do something that adds a little quality to your life, without complicating it anymore. It's always best to start small.

> **Where Does The Time Go?**
>
> Get up for work around 7.00am.
>
> Take a shower and get ready for work - 30 mins
>
> Wake son and make him breakfast - 30 mins
>
> Commute - 40 mins
>
> Work 9am to 5.20pm - 8 hrs 20 mins
>
> Eat lunch at my desk - 20 mins of social media
>
> Drive home via the store - 1 hr 20 mins
>
> Drive son to baseball - 20 mins
>
> Go to another couple of stores - 1 hr
>
> Pick son up and go home - 40 min round trip
>
> Make dinner - 20 mins
>
> Housework - 1 hr
>
> Watch TV - 1 hr
>
> Bed - 11pm
>
> **Time Spent On Work & Others?** 14 hrs 40 mins
>
> **Time Spent On Me?** 1 hr 20 mins

Susan's worksheet shows an average weekday when her son has after school activities. There are days when she does have fewer commitments which leaves her more time for herself, but all too often when she does have time for herself, she's too exhausted to do anything more than crash in front of the TV and chill with Netflix.

What I think this example shows is how little time people, especially parents, spend on themselves and their own wellbeing. If you look at Susan's time breakdown, the biggest part of her day is spent at work or sleeping, which I expect is the case for most people. However, the next biggest chunk of time is spent driving around. This can be a stressful activity and if we add that to the typical stresses of the workday, then her body could be experiencing elevated levels of cortisol even before she gets to work. Without getting much relief from an onslaught of cortisol, her blood sugar will stay elevated.

We can also see she does have an opportunity for lunch at work, but often she sits mindlessly in front of her computer looking at social media. When quizzed on this, Susan didn't have any work reason to sit at her desk eating lunch, it's just a habit.

What I'd like you to do now, is fill in your own timesheet. Once you've done that, we'll look at adding some self-care activities into your day.

If you want a Where Does the Time Go? worksheet, you can print a copy from my website drewcoster.com/worksheets

Self-Care Activities

Once we understand how many hours you spend in a day doing what you do, the first step is to figure out what self-care activities you can do for yourself. Let's forget about how much time you have or don't have for the moment, and let's look at some activities you used to enjoy, or still do. These are activities which rejuvenate you or give you a sense of happiness and wellbeing.

Take some time to think about these activities and write down at least two things under each time frame.

If I Had 10 Minutes I Could...?

This might be something like listening to music and dancing around the bedroom like no one's watching, taking a nap, playing with your cat or dog, or meditating.

If I Had 30 Minutes I Could...?

This might be something like reading a book, playing an instrument, drawing, going for a walk or practicing yoga.

If I Had 60 Minutes or More I Could...?

This might be something like exercising, taking a long bath, talking with a friend, hiking in the countryside or indulging in a full-body massage.

Now you've established some activities you like and how much time each activity takes, we need to figure out how to insert some of these activities into your day or week. If we go back to Susan's Where Does The Time Go? worksheet, it's clear she fills her day, so we don't have a lot of time to play with.

What is clear though is she can take a lunch break, but she doesn't do much with it. She also has a little time spare before bed.

Example Self-Care Changes

The first change I negotiated with Susan was to stop eating at her desk. We decided she would take her lunch and find a spot outside where she could eat. During this time, she'd also spend at least 20 minutes reading a book and not looking at social media.

Second, Susan goes to the store a lot, so we put a plan together for her to bulk cook meals on Sunday. Doing this will save her time on traveling to the store because she doesn't have anything ready at the end of the day when she's too tired to cook. Bulk cooking saves time when she's at her busiest. The plan was to bulk cook protein and roast vegetables and then portion out the meals to freeze. This way she has convenient food to hand when she's too busy or exhausted to cook.

This also negates the need for store-bought ready-meals, which we know are not the healthiest.

Susan used to practice yoga a few times a week until she just ran out of time. What we did was slowly add a 10-minute yoga workout into her day when she woke up. We decided slow yoga before her shower would not only help her get used to doing something enjoyable first thing in the morning but moving her body would be a wonderful way to wake up before her commute. These 10 minutes really didn't take much out of her morning, and in time she found she increased her practice until she did around 20-30 minutes of yoga (she also finally let her son make his own breakfast!).

The next change was in the car. Instead of listening to the radio in the car to and from work, she would listen to podcasts and audiobooks on topics she was interested in. Although this didn't change anything about her daily commute, she did use this time to start learning a new language because talking aloud in the car was easy to do.

The final change was to instigate a 'no TV in the bedroom' rule. Instead, Susan watched one of her shows on her tablet while she took a long bath before bed. This was a two-for-one activity which she looked forward to most nights.

As you can see, we really didn't do much to alter the time she had available, instead, we used her time more actively. What Susan discovered was small changes made significant improvements to how she felt during the day. Not only because she was spending a little more time on herself, but she also felt she could allow herself to have personal time without over complicating her already busy day.

I'm hoping you can see that even spending 10 minutes a day on your own self-care is often enough to give you a better sense of balance in the day. And if you have more time, then I would urge you to start thinking about what activity really recharges your batteries and support your journey toward cleansing your blood.

Weekly Action Plan

A weekly action plan builds on those behaviors you want to remind yourself to do on a daily, weekly or even monthly basis. It doesn't have to be comprehensive, more like a brief reminder of the tasks you want to focus on the most for that week. In my experience, those who flounder the most or feel overly challenged in the initial stages of the program, are those who don't invest time in pre-planning. Significant changes only happen when we invest time in repetition to build our new routines. Until those routines and choices become as automatic as our old behaviors, then we can lose our way without at least a basic plan.

Lifestyle change, overall, can go against everything you are familiar and comfortable with, which is why we're working to build a robust blueprint to help you keep on track. With a weekly action plan, you're not only working on changing some specific areas of your life, but the plan also acts as a visual aid in reminding you to keep working on certain tasks that are important to you.

Because our long-standing habits are choices which have been established over many months, years and even decades, it would be naïve to think we can just change those patterns overnight. It's just not realistic. And because we're beginning to challenge these ingrained habits, we need all the firepower we can create.

To undermine these old habits, we need to chip away at them day-by-day and your action plan is going to be a helpful weapon in winning this war of change.

The new tasks and behaviors you're learning are so new that when things get difficult, maybe you get tired or pushed for time, your old habits will come flying back and take over. However, in time, by following your meal plan, shopping list, and weekly action plan, your new behaviors will soon become as automatic as some of your old behaviors. With time and practice, you'll be eating, sleeping, exercising and relaxing in different ways than you used to do and that is ultimately going to help cleanse your blood.

Your plan doesn't have to be extensively detailed and the example below is really all you might need to keep certain tasks in the front of your mind. Even just a daily glance at your list will help to fix it into your brain.

- Be mindful of my all-or-nothing Thinking Traps.
- Make sure to eat every 3 hours.
- Drink 60oz of water before lunch.
- Add 10 mins of meditation after lunch.
- Bed by 9.30pm (turn the TV off!).
- Make sure to take snacks to work on Tue for long meeting.
- Plan Exception Eating meal for Saturday night.

I encourage clients to either set a calendar reminder that pops-up every day or write it on a Post-It and put it somewhere that you will see it multiple times a day. Visual reminders are powerful, but don't just look at your list - articulate! As I've said before, when you say something out loud it has more power than just a thought. Every day talk your way through your list.

The First Two Weeks

You're ready. You've done all your exercises. You've got a better idea of how you face change and all the things you need to do. You've got a plan of action and you're ready to go. Hopefully you're feeling confident about the changes you're about to make and the choices you've made so far. So, what about the beginning, what can you expect?

Personally, I think the first two weeks are often the hardest but once you get past those weeks, it gets a whole lot easier. In the beginning, when you're first kicking sugary food of choices out of your meal plans, there's going to be a physical consequence. I know not everyone will experience these physical symptoms when coming off sugar, but if you do, I want you to know these physical symptoms are temporary. No matter how terrible you feel, remind yourself, this too shall pass and when it does, you'll feel a whole lot better. Your blood will also thank you.

Here are the most common symptoms you might feel in the first week or two of coming off sugar.

Headaches and Dizziness

A dull headache that just seems to linger and doesn't go even after taking painkillers. You might also find your blood pressure jumps around and getting out of chairs can lead to dizziness.

Tiredness

You might feel as if your energy is just not there and everything seems like a struggle. Getting out of bed is hard. Walking and doing mundane tasks just feel like a grind.

Foggy Brain

You might find it hard to think clearly or be able to concentrate for any length of time.

Angry

You may find yourself getting angry at the smallest things. You may unexpectedly explode and find your anger is way out of proportion to whatever is going on.

Low Mood and Energy

Along with feeling tired, you may find your mood, and energy are significantly lower than normal. It can be hard to feel like doing any activity, even eating well. You might even feel sad and tearful at times. In extreme cases, you may find you don't want to get out of bed. Don't worry if this happens. Remember, this too shall pass.

Disturbed Sleep

You might find you are restless at night and find it hard to get to sleep and stay asleep for long. You also may wake up every couple of hours feeling hungry during the night and craving sugary snacks.

Flu-like Symptoms

Coming off carbs and sugar can lead to what is known as 'carb flu' or 'keto flu'. This is when you feel run down and have similar symptoms to a cold but without the runny nose and temperature. It's also usual for people to literally come down with a cold or flu as your body begins to detox from sugar.

Massive Cravings for Sugar

You'll start to see sugar everywhere. It's like the entire world suddenly becomes a donut, candy bar or bagel. Your brain will become your enemy, driving you, begging you to eat something sugary.

Aches and Pains

You might find your joints ache and you feel stiff all over.

Shakes and Sweats

This is more extreme, but people do get the shakes withdrawing from sugar. You might even feel hot and sweaty at times for no reason.

I know this all sounds bad, and you're unlikely to experience all these symptoms to their extremes but you might experience low levels of some, and that can feel uncomfortable. The good news is these symptoms usually fade after the first week. Low-grade headaches are typically the most common symptom, followed by cravings for sugar.

The problem with cravings is that as soon as you succumb to them and eat a sugar food, everything you went through in the last few days will be for nothing and you'll need to start withdrawing from it all over again. This can be extremely frustrating and is often the number one reason people give up early on any health related program where food is concerned.

Nobody wants to feel low and have to fight their own brain to keep control of their health but as I explained before, depending on your brain's reward loop, giving up sugar will be harder for some and easier for others. As tempting as the cravings may be, I really encourage you to face them with a steely resolve. Obviously, if you do feel incredibly unwell, always seek advice from your primary care physician.

The Second Week

Usually, by the second week, you'll start to feel brighter. You'll start to notice that you don't have any of the symptoms from the first week and your energy levels increase. Now, if you do still have the week one symptoms it doesn't necessarily mean you've done anything wrong because for a small number of people it can take two, three or even a month to get past the first week's symptoms. If you do still experience some of the symptoms, just take time to review the nutrition plan (coming up) again and compare it to what you have been eating. Sometimes you might be eating something you think is healthy but is full of sugar. I mostly see this with people who start eating a lot more fruit because they think it's healthy (pro tip: it's not). Many people go on a fruit binge when they start to give up sugar, but fruit is still sugar and needs to be eaten sparingly.

However, if your food is on point, and you're still having some symptoms this just shows how much your body is affected by sugar, and how carbohydrate-sensitive you are. If this sounds like you just keep working at getting healthy. Do everything you've planned to do and in time, you'll start to feel brighter and more energetic.

Once the symptoms have passed, the second and third week will feel like you're getting into your routine. If you're following your plan you should know what you are doing. Hopefully you'll have a house full of on-plan groceries and you're getting into a rhythm with eating every three hours. Again, don't worry if you're not there yet. Remember, baby steps are better than no steps. Even if you're doing one or two things well at this point, that's great. Just stick with it, because once you get into weeks three and four, you'll be doing great and feeling a whole lot better.

Maintenance Eating

Before we finish with this section, I want to talk about Maintenance Eating. This is an important step which is possibly several months ahead of you, but something I want you to be aware of even now.

The role of maintenance eating is to make sure you have a plan of how to eat well even after you've cleansed your blood. Getting healthy blood is just the middle phase of this program. Balancing your Five Pillars and keeping them balanced for the rest of your life is the ultimate goal (more about that soon, I promise).

The truth is, just because you work your butt off to cleanse your blood, it doesn't mean a thing if once you get clean, you go back to eating poorly again. Just because you cleanse your blood it doesn't mean it will magically stay clean for the rest of your life without continued vigilance and healthy lifestyle choices.

Time and again, I've seen people who get good blood results from their doctor and seemingly forget everything they'd learned and go back to eating unhealthily within six months to a year. It was like once they'd reached their goal, they figured they had everything under control and could relax. Exceptions became more routine.

The problem with that thinking is once you start to introduce more carbs and sugar back into your diet, you'll fire up your dopamine-loving brain again, and it will trick you into eating more from the NO food section. Instead of that once-a-week treat, it turns into a twice or more exceptions a week. Instead of a couple of slices of pizza on Saturday night, it becomes the entire pizza with four beers as a chaser.

So how do you manage maintenance eating? How do you find a happy medium between keeping your blood clean, while introducing a few foods you'd still like to enjoy but are not great for your blood?

To be honest, the easiest way is to just keep eating the way you would in the beginning of your program. Even when you start your program, there are no rigid restrictions, just certain things which are best avoided if possible. Treats and exceptions are encouraged, and you don't have to follow a fad diet for the rest of your life that is boring and unsustainable. Just keep your Five Pillars balanced and you'll have long-term success.

My hope for you is that your food choices won't really be an issue once you've cleansed your blood. Because if you've been eating well for six months to a year, you should be in a pretty good groove with the options you have, and you should be able to stay the course without the need to add anything from your old eating habits.

However good you are at sticking to your plan, I'd still like you to consider the questions below and write down your answers. Having a clear understanding of how you are going to approach the months at the end of your program will be invaluable in helping you stick to your long-term health plan. I also recommend referring to this worksheet regularly. Maybe set a calendar reminder to look at your answers at least once a month just to remind yourself of what your long-term goal is.

A worksheet for Maintenance Eating can be downloaded at drewcoster.com/worksheets

Maintenance Eating Questions

1. What have I learned about my past eating habits from this book?
2. What have I found most helpful by following this book to cleanse my blood?
3. What changes and improvements have I experienced since cleansing my blood?
4. How will I maintain these changes/improvements?
5. What support do I need to continue to do well?
6. What situations might trigger a setback in my maintenance?

7. What will I do to manage these setbacks and get back on track?
8. What are the signs that I'm falling back into old habits and not following my plan?
9. What action will I take if I notice I'm slipping back into old habits?
10. What are my goals for months 1-2?
11. What are my goals for months 3-6?
12. What are my goals for months 7-12?

Going Forward

By now, you'll have a clearer understanding of your change process, and how healthy thinking will be a big part of your success. Everything you've done so far will have raised your awareness of what it is you want to achieve and what roadblocks you might need to overcome.

It may sound strange, but don't underestimate the power of habitual thinking. The cliché of 'old habits die hard' is very true. Just because we become aware of our unhelpful thinking, it doesn't mean it will disappear overnight. Keep looking at your worksheets. Keep articulating what benefits you will gain from cleansing your blood, and don't forget to reframe negative thinking, even if it sounds silly in the beginning. Practice, practice, practice.

Over the next few sections I'll explain more about how to cleanse your blood and the practical steps you can take, but it will all be for nothing if your mindset isn't right. Honestly, the practicalities of cleansing your blood are straight forward. I'll give you all the information you will ever need to get well. However, only you can make the right choices for you. And if that annoying inner voice is still sabotaging, that practical advice is potentially worthless.

This is why I do encourage clients to take more time to work on understanding their thinking and the change process if this is an area where they typically struggle. There's no harm in waiting another week or two while practicing healthier thinking if it means you'll be more ready for change.

Right now, I have no doubt you will be successful if you take your time and don't forget to be kind to yourself. Be clear on what benefits you will gain from not having diabetes, prediabetes or metabolic syndrome. And remember slips, trips and falls are a healthy part of the process.

PART TWO:

FIVE PILLARS

"The Critical part of a balance in life is choosing priorities."
- Byron Pulsifer

Five Pillars of Good Health

As a complex human there are many awe-inspiring functions which go into making your body perform properly. So far, we've looked at the mind, emotion and behavior connection to lifestyle change, and now it's important to understand how the physical self needs supporting too. For my clients, I find it's extremely important for them to understand that no one decision or food choice is going to cleanse your blood. To make successful change it is all about balancing all Five Pillars of Good Health.

As much as media and other books suggest that eating better and exercising is the way to change your health, these are only a part of what will really reverse your condition. And in truth, focusing on just those two things will often have an adverse effect to your blood condition. With all this information on food and exercise available, you'd be forgiven for thinking that they are the most important things to focus on, but that is often furthest from the truth. Real change will come from understanding and balancing five, not just two Pillars to Good Health.

These Five Pillars in order of importance are: sleep, water, nutrition, stress and exercise. Each Pillar has its place in your overall health system, and ultimately, we want them all to be balanced and functioning well. However, as part of my approach is progress not perfection, there are three Pillars I think are essential to focus on first. These three Pillars will also give you the most bang for your buck, regarding how quickly and efficiently you can reverse your condition.

The essential Pillars of Good Health are sleep, then water and then nutrition. That's the order of success. Because I say these are essentials, this doesn't mean we neglect the other two important Pillars.

I do suggest putting more effort into each Pillar sequentially, while also working on the others. What I mean by this is focus more on sleep than any other Pillar until this one improves significantly, then focus more on the next Pillar water. While all the time still working on the others, but maybe not with as much focus.

The reason for this is we often like to tackle the things we think are the easiest or what we like best. If you focus more on nutrition but don't sort bad sleep out, your food choices are not going to make a whole lot of difference. But if you switch that up, and get your sleep straight first, your nutrition will be lot more effective.

I also like people to be comfortable with the change they are making to one Pillar before moving on to the next. This might mean the process of change is a little slower, but you will be setting yourself up to be more successful long-term.

Because I think making sleep your priority to start with, over the next few pages I will explain how you can get better quality sleep and overcome any challenges you might have. Once sleep is good, move on to the next Pillar and then the next.

When all your essential Pillars are in balance, then it's time to continue to the next two supporting Pillars of stress and exercise. I know what you're thinking: "Exercises is last on this priority list and is not essential?" Correct, it's not essential. Which is why many people who jump in and try to cleanse their blood or lose weight through the exercise Pillars first, often fail quickly. Don't get me wrong, some exercise is important (not as much as you think), but in the beginning of your program, it doesn't need to be a priority.

In fact, if we look at how the human body survives in respect to these Pillars, you'll get a rough idea of why the Pillars are in the order they are.

Without Sleep

We become delirious after three to four days. Research on rats shows them dying after two weeks of no sleep. Sleep is the essential and most often overlooked Pillar on our list.

Without Water

We can die after eight to ten days (three days in harsher conditions such as desert or extreme cold).

Without Food

We can die after around three weeks of starvation.

With Stress

We can continue to live with chronic stress, although eventually it can lead to psychological and physiological problems, but this might be after a matter of years.

Without Exercise

We'll continue to live relatively fine. It may reduce our life expectancy somewhat and the quality of our physical ability will be impaired, but you can survive without exercise. Take the amazing Stephen Hawking as an extreme example.

Earlier I said consistency is the key to reversing your condition, and that is true. Where you want to apply that consistency is with balancing the Five Pillars to Good Health. This is where you will find your long-term success in reversing your condition.

Five Pillars Exercise

Understanding how balanced your Pillars are will give you a sense of where you are in the process of overall good health. Over the next few pages I will talk about how much water and sleep etc. You will need to be in balance, but right now, this exercise is just to give you a sense of how balanced your health is right now.

Take a moment to mark on these Pillars where you think you currently are in terms of balance in any typical day.

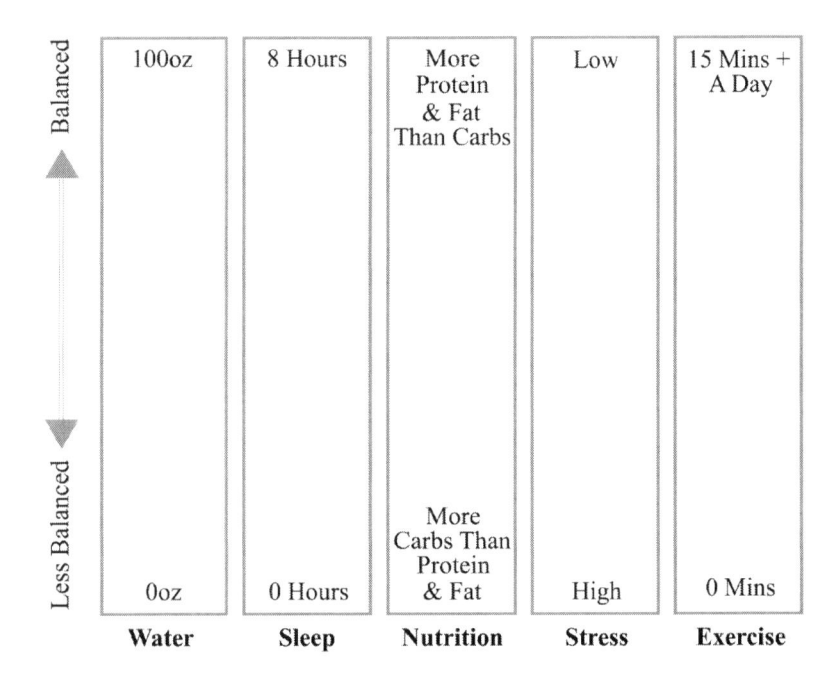

	Water	Sleep	Nutrition	Stress	Exercise
Balanced	100oz	8 Hours	More Protein & Fat Than Carbs	Low	15 Mins + A Day
Less Balanced	0oz	0 Hours	More Carbs Than Protein & Fat	High	0 Mins

Now you have this information, we'll work on them in a step-by-step way. Once all Pillars are balanced, you'll find you've achieved your goal of reversing your condition. It really is as simple as that.

If you want a Five Pillars worksheet, you can print a copy from my website drewcoster.com/worksheets

Pillar #1: Sleep

You may find it strange to prioritize sleep as the first of the Five Pillars, but there really are several major health reasons for getting enough sleep. Good mental health is the main reason, but good sleep is even more essential with your condition. The reason for this is that a lack of sleep boosts your sympathetic nervous system (your fight, flight or freeze function) and this system activates a hormone called Cortisol. And one of the main functions of Cortisol is to raise your glucose levels. That's right, by not sleeping, your glucose levels which are elevated anyway with your condition, become even higher naturally.

Plus, the kicker is, your body will become even more insulin resistant just from sleeping poorly. So, not only might you be producing more glucose when you eat, but your body is raising it for you because you might be lacking quality sleep.

Seems unfair, right? Well, if you've ever wondered why you have your condition despite eating well and exercising often, it's highly likely that you aren't sleeping well enough, and this is creating a negative health cycle. If you need more information on why you really have your condition, take a look at the **Your Blood** section in this book.

If you find sleep isn't an issue, and you are getting close to 8 hours a night, then you can skip ahead to the Water section if you wish. But if you find getting enough sleep or getting quality sleep is a challenge, here are some of my top strategies for getting more sleep.

Strategies for Getting More Sleep

We covered the importance of sleep as one of the essential Five Pillars of Good Health, so now I want to go through some of the common issues and solutions you can employ to help you get better sleep. From what was covered earlier, it's my belief that poor sleep is the catalyst for why so many people have a blood condition.

Poor sleep patterns don't only lead to diabetes, prediabetes, and metabolic syndrome but also mental health issues like depression and anxiety. These problems arise mainly because tiredness affects how two important hormones leptin, and ghrelin work. These are covered extensively in the **Your Blood** section if you're not up to speed on them, but we know from research that when these hunger hormones are messed up, the effect on our insulin and blood sugar levels are exaggerated.

Studies have shown that if you go a single night without more than six hours of sleep, then you're more likely to want to eat more the following day. Not only will you eat more food but you're more likely to eat snacks to get enough energy to function. And as snacks tend to be full of sugar this gives you that quick boost of energy your brain craves when you're tired.[87,88]

If you are a chronically bad sleeper or don't get enough sleep at night for whatever reason, it's will be harder for you to eat healthily. Therefore, I really encourage you to try and make sleep a priority. It won't make much difference if you make changes to your nutrition if you haven't got a handle on sleep first. Because even if you are eating well, poor sleep is going to sabotage your progress because of the higher levels of Cortisol and the dysfunctional leptin and ghrelin hormones.

Sleep Problem #1: Obstructive Sleep Apnea (OSA)

Sleep Apnea (or Obstructive Sleep Apnea for its full title) is a problem a lot of people with diabetes have, especially if they are overweight. But OSA can also be due to having a large tongue or tonsils; even the shape of your head and neck can have an effect. Also, being over 40 years old does increase your chances of having OSA. It's common not to be aware you have sleep apnea, so if you go through this list and recognize you have a few of the signs of sleep apnea, it might be time to talk to your doctor.

Sleep apnea happens when the walls of the throat relax and narrow during sleep, even sometimes collapsing altogether to cut off your airway. OSA is typically diagnosed when your breathing is observed to stop for at least 10 seconds while you sleep. Think about that and try this experiment. Expel all the air from your lungs and wait 10 seconds before you take a breath. 10 seconds is a long time, and it doesn't feel good. With OSA you could be doing this repeatedly through the night which can lead to some serious long-term effects on your body and mind.

When you stop breathing, your body does have a mechanism to wake you up to breathe, usually with an audible gasp. After that you'll tend to go back to sleep with no memory of waking and not breathing. If you sleep with a partner, they might notice you thrashing or gasping, and it can be quite distressing to witness.

I worked with a woman who got so anxious about her husband not breathing in the night that she used to stay awake to make sure he was okay. Sadly, the effect of this was that she became seriously anxious, fatigued and depressed until finally needing hospitalization. OSA is very serious and doesn't only affect the person who suffers from it.

This action of breathing being restricted, and your body waking to breathe and then falling back to sleep can happen multiple times in a night, and in severe cases, every minute or two. Severe sleep apnea can lead to many physical and psychological problems, including weight gain, high blood pressure, and constant fatigue during the day. Even mild sleep apnea can have a devastating effect on how you function.

Signs You Might Have OSA

Snoring and Gasping

It can be true that if you snore, you don't necessarily have sleep apnea. Most of us at one time or another will snore when we sleep, and this can be just simple snoring or primary snoring. This is where there is partial blockage anywhere in the throat which can be down to the angle of the head when we sleep. Sleep apnea snoring is often a louder and more frequent type of snoring, often punctuated with no breathing for a few seconds, followed by some snorting, gasping or choking.

Frequent Dry Mouth in the Morning

Waking up with a dry mouth isn't that comfortable but it isn't life-threatening, either. However, it could be a sign that you have sleep apnea. In fact, people with sleep apnea are twice as likely to experience dry mouth than people without it.

Constant Daytime Fatigue, Depression and Irritability

We know from studies that if your REM sleep is interrupted for one or two nights then your mood and cognitive functioning will become impaired. When you stop breathing with sleep apnea and wake up gasping for breath, it's this action which interrupts your REM sleep cycle; and without that cycle, you won't have the refreshing restorative sleep you need to be able to function well. If you have sleep apnea, especially if you have moments of not breathing, you'll be taken out of REM sleep each time you wake up. Poor sleep cycles can lead to chronic fatigue, cognitive impairment and can eventually lead to many mood disorders, especially depression.

Increased Hunger During the Day

As mentioned at the start of this chapter, when you go for a couple of nights without quality sleep your brain's way to compensate for the lack of energy is to encourage you to eat simple carbs and sugars like chocolate, chips, soda or cookies. These sugars give you a temporary boost in mood and energy, but within 10-15 minutes, the blood sugar spike you got from the food is over, and your blood sugar will drop, leading to more fatigue. This is a cycle that leads to more and more health problems. Clearly, the lack of restorative sleep plus the addition of more carbs into your diet is one of the main reason's diabetes, prediabetes, and metabolic syndrome are on the rise.

Acid Reflux or Heartburn

Research isn't entirely clear why this is, but people with OSA are more prone to acid reflux, which is also known as Gastroesophageal Reflux (GERD). Around 75% of people diagnosed with OSA will wake from their sleep with acid reflux. However, what researchers aren't clear on is whether OSA leads to GERD or whether GERD leads to OSA. Either way, changes in airway pressure from OSA can lead you to develop acid reflux whether or not you've been diagnosed with GERD.

Nocturnal Teeth Grinding (Sleep Bruxism)

If you wake with jaw pain, or you often grind your teeth when you sleep, you're not alone. Around one in four people with sleep apnea grind their teeth. The exact reason for this behavior is not known, but a combination of anxiety, fatigue and sleep apnea mean you're more likely to do this.

Solution to Obstructive Sleep Apnea

The best and only real solution to OSA is to go to your doctor and get a referral to a sleep study, as they'll be able to diagnose your issue and arrange for you to get the right treatment. This treatment might be in the form of a Continuous Positive Airway Pressure Device (CPAP) which is a mask that goes on your face to deliver the right amount of air pressure while you sleep to keep your airway open. This might sound worse than it is, but a CPAP can make an amazing difference to your sleep and overall well-being.

The type of CPAP many clients seem to get on with is called a Nasal Pillow, which is a CPAP that just fits over the nose, leaving the mouth uncovered.

Typically, clients who stick with a CPAP generally do amazingly well cleansing their blood and report having a lot more energy and clarity of thinking than they did before the CPAP. Those who try it but don't stick with it tend to continue struggling with their program because they still don't get quality sleep.

The other types of treatment for OSA are things like getting a dental appliance fitted which sits in your mouth while you sleep to reposition the lower jaw and tongue. This increases the airway opening in the back of the throat which can sometimes be enough to help you sleep better.

The last treatment type is surgery. This is often done to remove excess tissue from your airway to help you breathe better.

One tip when talking to your doctor about OSA is to make sure you take your own log of how poorly you sleep and a record of your energy levels from the last month. Logging your own OSA can be tricky but a gadget like the Fitbit is quite good at recognizing movement when you sleep, and one of the signs of OSA is a lot movement during sleep as your body responds to not getting enough oxygen.

Sleep Problem #2: Watching TV in the Bedroom

Having a TV in the bedroom is too tempting. It's all too easy to go to bed, switch the TV on and watch just one more show. Having a TV on in the bedroom encourages the brain to stay active, and the images and sound will stimulate the brain, making it harder to fall asleep.

Our body has a natural sleep system called the circadian rhythm, and this rhythm is controlled by the hormones Melatonin and Cortisol. Melatonin is the hormone which kicks in as night approaches, and it's the hormone that makes us feel sleepy. Now, cortisol does the opposite. As daybreak approaches, the Cortisol hormone rises, and we start to wake up.

Having a bright room will affect sleep very much. What researchers have found is that blue light emitted from TV's and other electronic screens is a lot stronger and suppresses the release of melatonin. This means anything that emits a blue light is bad news for natural sleep patterns. Therefore, at the time that your body is trying to slow you down and get you to sleep, the blue light shining in your eyes from your TV is telling your body that it's still daytime and you need to stay awake. As you can imagine, this is confusing to your hormones and is a no-win situation for your body. Not only do you drive yourself to stay up later to watch a show but you're confusing the signals your body is receiving – whether to stay awake or fall asleep. Long-term watching of TV at night will interfere with natural melatonin release to the point that it switches off and you'll find it harder and harder to fall asleep naturally.

Some people tell me they find falling asleep in front of the TV helps, but the reality is they more than likely fall asleep from exhaustion potentially hours after they ought to have fallen asleep to get a solid 6-8 hours.

By stimulating the brain this late at night and interfering with your circadian rhythm you are delaying your body's ability to go into REM sleep. This is the deep-interval sleep when you dream, which is linked to the restorative aspects of sleep. Without REM sleep you can become increasingly tired during the day, and this low energy will lead to the desire for more carbs and sugar food to help give the brain more energy to keep you awake.

Fatigue from Lack of REM Sleep

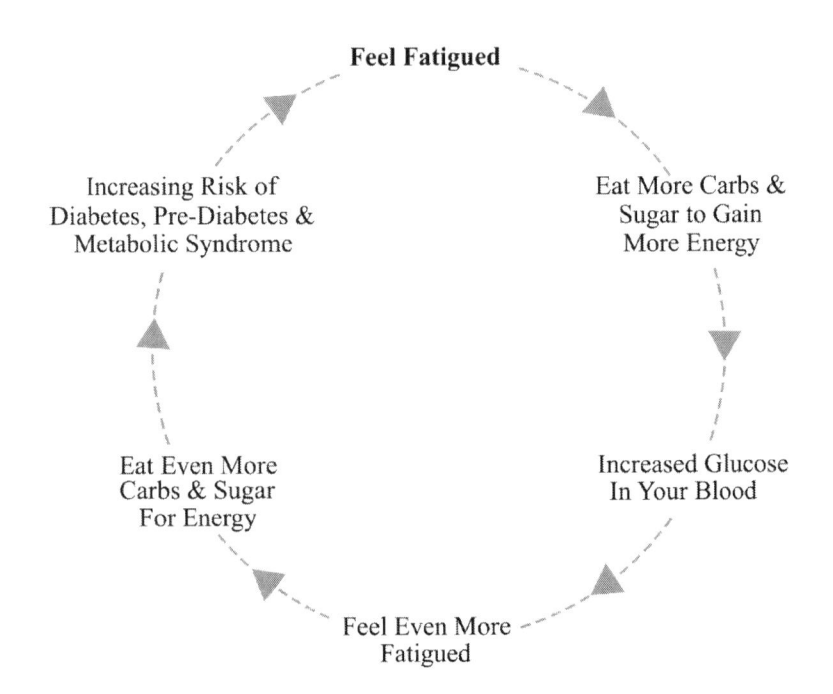

Feel Fatigued → Eat More Carbs & Sugar to Gain More Energy → Increased Glucose In Your Blood → Feel Even More Fatigued → Eat Even More Carbs & Sugar For Energy → Increasing Risk of Diabetes, Pre-Diabetes & Metabolic Syndrome → Feel Fatigued

A Harvard study also showed that the more our sleep is affected, the more blood sugar levels increase, and our leptin levels go down. So, knowing what you know about how your hormones are affected by insulin and blood sugar, you can see where this is all going, right? It's clear that watching TV at night doesn't only stop you from falling asleep easily but also encourages the body to break down, increasing or creating your condition, even if you've been eating well and exercising regularly. When our circadian rhythm becomes interrupted many people start to take another inhibitor of good sleep, and that's sleep aids (we'll cover that in a moment).

Solution to Watching TV in the Bedroom

First and foremost, the best solution is to remove the TV from the bedroom. I know what you'll say: *"But I'll just stay up and watch TV in another room instead, and not be in bed."* My answer to that is, if you want to get well and reverse your condition, then some self-control is inevitable. You need to see sleep as a treat rather than something that is tearing you away from a TV show you've probably seen before (or can DVR). Better sleep is setting yourself up for long-term success. I suggest not watching TV 30-60 minutes before bed to give your hormones time to move you towards sleep.

Sleep Problem #3: Using Phones or Tablets in Bed

Just as TV's emit blue light, so do smartphones, tablets and other electronic equipment, so the same advice for TV watching goes for all electronics.

These days, many people sit in bed checking Facebook, email, news, or just reading an eBook on their equipment but as we've learned, anything with blue light will affect our sleep patterns negatively. Also, many social apps like Facebook, Instagram and YouTube are designed to keep you engaged for as long as possible, so thinking that you'll just spend a few mindless minutes on those apps is not going to happen. I know I've gone onto YouTube to watch one thing and found that I'm still on it an hour or two later watching kittens playing the piano.

Smartphones and tablets have become both a blessing and a curse, and I think it's a smart idea to take all electronics out of the bedroom if you have a problem with staying up late using these devices. Just like removing the TV, if you don't have it near you, you won't engage with it. If you do a have an issue with using electronics in bed, here are a few solutions to make that less problematic to you getting better sleep.

Solution to Using Smartphones or Tablets in Bed

On most iPhones, iPads and Android phones there are blue light filters built in which you can turn on. If I know I'm aiming to go to bed around 9.30pm, then I'll make sure my blue light filter automatically comes on around 8.30pm to make sure I'm not having any blue light interfere with my melatonin release.

When I read in bed, I use the Amazon Kindle Paperwhite. Now, this also has small LED lights in the device, which do emit blue light, but what I have found with this device is that as the device is backlit, and the light is designed to shine onto the screen and away from the eyes, there's less impact on my brain. My experience is in no way scientific, but I find the Kindle Paperwhite to be a good compromise to having a bright light shining into my eyes or having a bedside lamp on, so I can read a paper book (plus, the light disturbs my wife if she's sleeping).

How to Turn on Blue Light Filters

iPhone & iPad

Got to Settings >Display & Brightness > Night Shift. From there you can set the time you want the filter to work. You can also set the color temperature of your screen. What this means is that the blue light is replaced with a red light which doesn't affect sleep. You'll find that your screen has an orange hue to it, which is also how you'll know the filter is on.

Google Pixel

Not all Android phones have Night Mode as of update 7.1.1. If you have a Pixel phone, then you have Night Mode installed and to access this you go to Settings > Display > Night Light. From there you can set the time you want the filter to work and just like the iPhone, you can also set the color temperature of your screen.

Samsung Galaxy Device

Samsung version of Android is a little different. To active the night mode you go to Settings > Display > Blue Light Filter. Again, you can set a custom time when you want this to turn on at night.

Android Other

For those who have other Android devices, you'll need to install a third-party app. There are several on the Play Store and you can search by just typing Blue Light Filters. The one I like is called Twilight by Urbandroid Team, but feel free to try a few out.

Sleep Problem #4: Environment

I'm going to assume you've removed the TV from your bedroom, so the next thing we need to get in order is making sure the room is dark enough, cool enough and devoid of distracting noises. Making sure you have a consistent environment for sleep is essential. When you sleep, if the room isn't dark enough, when you're in the light-sleep phase of your sleep cycle it can be easy to wake, and more difficult to fall back to sleep with a bright room versus a dark room.

Alternatively, if the room is too warm or too cold, you can also wake and find it harder to fall back to sleep. And if there is a lot of noise that will also alert the brain and waking up will be common.

One way to think of your bedroom is like a cave. A cave is in our DNA and a cool, dark, safe place to sleep and that's how our bedroom should be. We may have evolved from our ancestors, but some things are hardwired into us, and being comfortable and safe while sleeping is still essential to good sleep.

Solution to Increasing Comfort

Most sleep experts recommend having the bedroom temperature set between 65 and 72 degrees. Personally, I like the temperature around 68-70 and I also use an overhead fan to move the air around the room. I really don't sleep well when I get too hot or the air becomes stuffy, so if you're able to change the thermometer in that room, experiment with different temperatures until you find the ideal one for you.

The other thing to consider is having a mattress and pillow that doesn't get too hot and make you sweat. Memory foam pillows and mattresses are comfortable because they conform to your body, however, they can also keep the heat in around you which can lead to sweating and feeling overheated. This will again lead to wakefulness through the night as you struggle to keep cool.

If you're in a room that is slightly noisy - maybe your partner snores (which is common), then you might want to think about wearing earplugs to bed. Some people are reluctant to wear them, thinking they won't hear their alarm clock or other noises in the house but in my experience, this isn't the case. Earplugs take some of the noise away but you're still able to hear alarms, and even some snoring but it just takes that edge off that allows the brain to be less disturbed by noise during the night. There are many assorted brands and sizes of earplugs, so try a few different ones and change them regularly to avoid any risk of ear infections.

As well as temperature and noise, darkness is a big deal. If you find your room is too bright from outside light, you could try blackout curtains to negate most of this light. I personally like the darkest room possible, but my wife prefers it lighter; our compromise is that I wear an eye-mask at night if the moon is too bright. In fact, a recent study on the effects of wearing earplugs and eye masks for increasing REM sleep in a bright and noisy ICU unit showed they helped to promote better sleep by raising melatonin levels naturally.[94]

Earplugs and eye masks are cheap and easy to get hold of from most large grocery stores, pharmacies or online. I recommend giving them a chance.

Sleep Problem #5: Waking to go to the Bathroom

It's quite normal to wake to pee during the night (known as nocturia or nocturnal polyuria) if you have diabetes because high blood glucose leads to more urination. If you find you are waking every three hours or less then it might be worth getting checked out by your doctor because peeing at night can also be a symptom of other problems such as a bladder infection, an enlarged prostate, incomplete urine emptying condition, or hormone changes for women.

Solutions to Waking to go to the Bathroom

I'll cover water intake a little later but for now, just know that water is essential to the body. It's best not to be afraid to drink just because you pee a lot because peeing is what you want to happen as it's partly how your body gets rid of toxins. However, peeing at night can be very disruptive, so do some of the following to avoid unnecessary trips to the bathroom.

Reduce coffee and alcohol use, especially at night. Don't drink coffee or alcohol within six hours of going to bed. I know many people use alcohol to help them sleep but just because alcohol may help you fall asleep, it will limit your REM sleep, and this will again interfere with good sleep. The other thing about alcohol and coffee is that they are also diuretics and cause your body to produce more urine, which, if you're drinking late at night will probably lead to you waking up to pee.

The other thing I suggest is to stop drinking water or any liquids about two hours before bed just to let any urine in your system flush through.

If you are on medication for high blood pressure this too can make you want to pee more, especially if you take it at night. There's not a lot you can do about this for now but soon enough, when you've cleaned your blood, you'll hopefully not need those pills anymore and you should sleep better.

Sleep Problem #6: Racing Mind

Many people I've worked with are very conscientious and have a lot going on in their lives. They often work extremely hard and like to do a good and thorough job in everything they're involved with. It's a great trait to have a strong work ethic and a desire to do good. However, the downside to this is that often they bring work home with them and find it difficult to slow their brain down, thinking about all they need to do at work the next day. They think about the plans, the meetings, the tasks ahead – and all this information whirls around and around.

While this is going on the brain needs to stay active by thinking, remembering and problem-solving. Not only does this exhaust the brain because it doesn't get any downtime, it also means your brain considers what you are thinking about is important. And when something is important, the brain creates more space in our 'thinking brain' to spend on these problems.

If you've ever gone to bed with something on your mind, you've probably experienced how the brain just churns this information over and over, and no matter how much you want to sleep, it keeps going over conversations you had or need to have. It goes over emails you need to write or people you need to reach out to. But it doesn't just do that once, it goes over the information time and again just because it is trying to remember all the things it needs to do when it's tired and doesn't really have the capacity to do what is asked of it. So, out of anxiety of forgetting it goes around and around all the time, making it harder for you to switch off and go to sleep.

Solution to Racing Mind

There are two things you can do to get your racing mind to calm down. First, you take 10 minutes just before getting ready for bed, to sit down with a notepad and spend that 10 minutes thinking about all the things that are on your mind. You then jot these thoughts down on the pad. Once you've done that, here's the secret to making this transfer from thoughts onto paper more effective; you have to verbally articulate what you are thinking out loud and say what you've written down.

Just as I discussed earlier in the book about articulating our thoughts out loud to make them carry more emotional weight, using this technique here does the same thing. What this does is take a thought and make it more real; because by saying the issue out loud your brain hears you and it will not only remember what you are saying but it also acts on what you are saying. For example, I might write down and say: *"I need to make sure I wake up early tomorrow as I have a meeting with my boss at 8.30."* When we think about something that is causing us some underlying anxiety, then our fear of not waking up on time can lead us to worry about waking up, therefore our brain doesn't rest at night because it is worrying about not waking up. What happens next is your brain will have you waking up every hour to check that you haven't missed your alarm.

By doing this anxiety routine, you're not sleeping, and you won't be your best when you finally do go to work. Now, if you struggle with recurring thoughts at night, this task of writing things down and articulating them will turn your concern into a 'solution statement'. You can do something like this: *"I will wake up early tomorrow as I have a meeting with my boss. I know I will wake when I hear my alarm and I'll be refreshed and ready to go, with no concerns."*

Right here, you've taken your concern out of your head and told your brain it can relax because you know you'll be fine in the morning. Believe it or not, as your brain hears this statement it's very likely to relax. I know I've asked you to say things out loud a lot throughout this book and that's because verbal articulation, whenever you have a problem, will always be more helpful than just thinking something internally. Give it a go.

Sleep Problem #7: Using Sleep Aids for Sleep

Just as some people use alcohol as a sleep aid, there are also prescription or over-the-counter sleep aids which for occasional use may be helpful, but long-term use will have the opposite effect to what you hoped for. Drugs like Ambien (Zolpidem), which is the most popular prescription sleeping drug, does have a lot of side-effects that can affect you more than it will help. Some of the common side-effects are drowsiness during the day (which clearly is the opposite of we want), headaches, a stuffed or runny nose, memory loss, body and muscle aches.

I understand that when you're having trouble falling asleep, it seems easier to pop a pill, and I am one of those people who occasionally takes an Ambien but never more than once a month. The problem comes when we start using sleep aids as a daily quick fix.

These tablets lose their effectiveness the longer you take them, and in time you may find your dose going up and up to be effective. This leads to more and more side-effects and less chance you'll be able to reverse your condition without a struggle.

One more thing about hypnotics (as they are known), they also switch off your own circadian rhythm, so once you stop taking them, you may find falling asleep becomes even harder than it was before you took them. This then can lead to this type of vicious cycle.

Cycle of Poor Sleep on Sleeping Aides

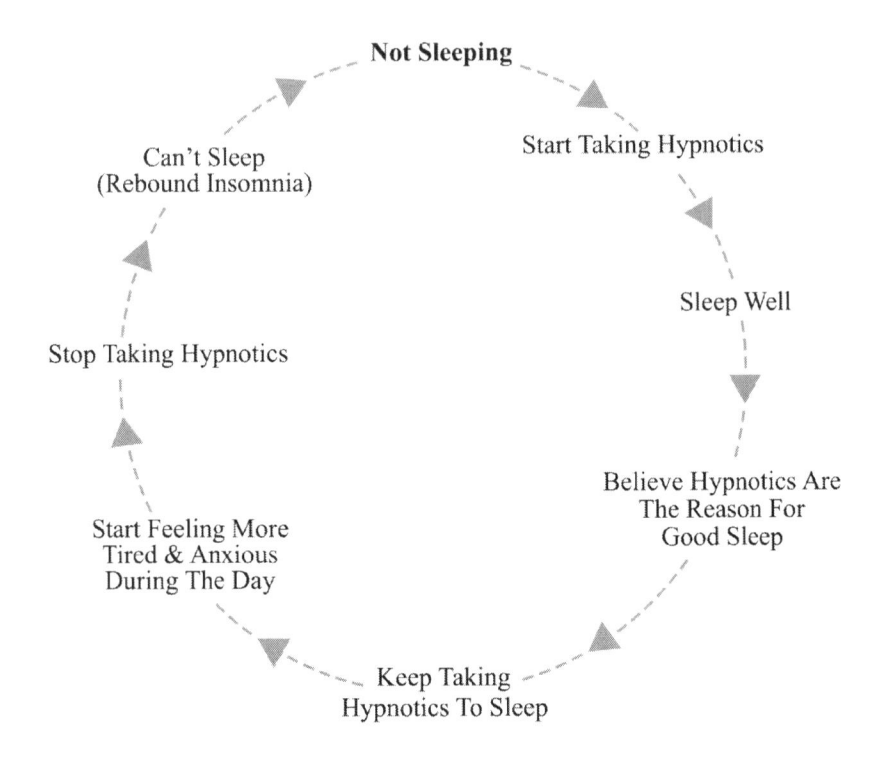

```
                    Not Sleeping
         Can't Sleep              Start Taking Hypnotics
       (Rebound Insomnia)

                                        Sleep Well

       Stop Taking Hypnotics

                                   Believe Hypnotics Are
                                      The Reason For
                                        Good Sleep
       Start Feeling More
         Tired & Anxious
         During The Day
                       Keep Taking
                      Hypnotics To Sleep
```

These cycle and sleep problems can also happen when using over-the-counter products like ZzzQuil. ZzzQuil's main ingredient is diphenhydramine, which is the active ingredient in the antihistamine, Benadryl. In fact, ZzzQuil has double the diphenhydramine of Benadryl which is why you feel sleepy when taking these tablets. However, just like prescription drugs, you'll soon develop a resistance to the over-the-counter sleep aids and again, you might start taking more to get any effect from them, or you might progress to prescription drugs without fixing everything else in this sleep list first.

Where possible, I would encourage you to *not* take sleeping aids on a regular basis. Getting back into your own circadian rhythm and allowing your body to produce its own melatonin might take a few weeks but that is ultimately healthier for you than getting stuck in a rut using medication for sleep.

Solutions to Reducing Sleep Aids

Most doctors would agree, the occasional use of sleep aids isn't a problem but if you find you're taking them multiple times a week, then you are creating more sleep problems for yourself later.

If you have a problem sleeping for a week or two, it's best to first see your doctor, as there may be other issues occurring that they can address. Other than that, go through all these sleep problems and solutions and make sure you've addressed them all first, as any time you can fix a health problem in the most natural way possible, the better off you and your health will be.

Sleep Problem #8: Eating Carbs Before Bed

I encourage people to eat just before bed but where the real problem comes is *what* is eaten before bed. The message for years has been to not eat before bed, and I think a lot of people still think of that as an absolute law, but it really isn't. There are certain things which are best avoided before bed, and I know many clients who feel hungry before bed but fight that urge to eat. They end up going to bed on an empty stomach (which is not ideal), or they'll eat some cereal to beat their hunger.

The problem with choices like cereal is they contain so much sugar and carbs that they will create glucose energy in your body – and having energy in your blood before you go to sleep is not the ideal way to increase quality sleep. If you eat carbs at night, you'll find yourself in a situation where your body is trying to slow down and sleep, but your metabolism is ramping up to deal with all the sugar you've ingested.

Essentially, you're stoking the fire at the exact time you want it to go out. Because of this energy release, you might find you become restless in bed. You might start tossing and turning with your mind firing off thoughts about subjects that aren't relevant at this time of night. You might also start to get angry because you're not getting to sleep, and this begins driving anxiety thinking about being tired and not functioning the next day. Of course, all of this leads to a poor night's sleep; which can sadly lead to the desperation of reaching for sleep aids.

Solution to Eating Less Carbs Before Bed

A good rule of thumb is to not eat carbs within 2 hours of going to bed. Sometimes that's unavoidable but as a daily plan, try and make sure you give your body a little space to process any carbohydrates you might have eaten while still allowing time for your body to naturally start slowing down before bed.

I talk about meal timing in the **Nutrition** section, and I always recommend having some form of fat before going to bed; such as almond butter about 30 minutes before bed. The reason for this is two-fold. First, fat is slow to digest and can help feed you slowly through the night, which can limit a drop in your blood sugar which may lead to you waking during the night and feeling hungry.

The other reason is that it's a tasty treat, and it's something to look forward to in the bedtime process. A lot of people want something sweet as a dessert after dinner but as we're trying to avoid sweet things, that's not a clever idea. However, if you know in a couple of hours you can have some delicious peanut or almond butter, then that encourages people not to dip into snacks before bed.

For those of you who do not like almond or peanut butter, you can have some plain Greek yogurt or even some cheese, like mozzarella or half an avocado. It doesn't really matter what you choose to eat before bed if it is mostly fat and contains little to no carbs.

Napping During the Day

I'm an advocate of napping during the day. I love a good afternoon nap and I find it does give me energy for the next phase of the afternoon. When I used to work in a psychiatric hospital, I would make sure I left myself a good 10 minutes at the end of my lunch break to get in a power nap which would set me up for the rest of the afternoon (self-care!). However, there is a difference between naps and sleeping.

For me, a nap is something that doesn't last longer than 15 minutes. To make sure I keep to that time I set my alarm for 10-15 minutes and I close my eyes and rest. I've done this for years, and it works for me, but I know that doesn't mean it will necessarily work for you. It also doesn't mean I will sleep for that length of time. I might be awake but just resting; and closing my eyes can be just as helpful.

In many ways you could replace a nap for meditation, as they do the same thing – they give your brain a mini-break. Some people feel worse after a short nap, and if that is you, mediation is probably the better way to go.

If you do find napping difficult, you might be more like my wife. When she has a nap, it can last two hours, and although she feels great when she wakes up, this isn't something you can generally do during your working day. Sleeping too long during the day can also mess up your sleep patterns at night, often making it much harder to go to sleep at a reasonable time or making it harder to sleep through the night and getting your 6-8 hours. If your bedtime is usually around 9 pm and you sleep for an hour or two during the day, you might find that bedtime gets pushed back by a few hours, which eats into how long you can sleep for.

A lot of people with your condition also get home from work feeling exhausted and have a nap as soon as they sit down. I'm not as keen on this type of nap, even if it is for 10 minutes, as napping in the evening can also interfere with getting to sleep later. If you come home tired, it's most likely due to your nutrition for the day not being on point or maybe you're not sleeping well at night and your body has used up all your energy to keep you functioning.

If you do find you're an after-work napper, then look at your nutrition during the day and make sure you are eating enough every 3 hours. Also, if you can, see if you can nap at lunchtime instead. Ideally, if you follow this information, you should start to have more energy throughout the day naturally, and you might not need to nap at all.

Solution to Make Sure Your Naps are Awesome

As I mentioned, if you have a nap, make sure that it is nearer the middle of the day, rather than in the evening. Also set an alarm to wake you in no later than 15 minutes after closing your eyes. Even if you don't nap, just resting for a short period can still be beneficial.

Some people like to meditate, and this does a similar thing. Ten minutes of meditating is like a mini-vacation for your brain. You don't have to nap to get the benefits of just taking some time out to let your brain have downtime.

Pillar #2: Water

Before we look at the importance of water, let's talk about one of the hidden heroes of good health -- minerals. If you read any magazine article about losing weight and being healthy, you'll read a lot about how to burn belly fat and get buns of steel, but they certainly don't talk about the immense importance of minerals.

Yes, minerals. These are the forgotten, and often ignored cousins to vitamins. Many people make sure they get enough vitamins or protein during the day, but minerals are not on most people's radar.

The easiest way to imagine what minerals do is to think of a brick wall. Now imagine that proteins are the bricks, which are strong and sturdy. Now imagine you're building a house out of brick. You take each brick and you place it on top of the other. Up and up it goes. From a distance it might look impressive, but if you push any of the bricks that wall will collapse. Why? Because they don't have any mortar to fix them together.

If proteins are like bricks, minerals are the mortar. Without a balance of minerals, your entire system won't be strong and can easily come crushing down, no matter how good the exterior looks. That's how important minerals are.

Another reason why water and minerals are so important is when you change the way you eat and focus on reducing carbohydrates and remove processed food to cleanse your blood, your body will use water and minerals differently than before. Instead of retaining water and minerals when eating poorly (think bloating and swelling in your body), on a better-balanced diet of low-to-moderate carbs the body will be expelling more water and minerals. Which means, if you don't have a good balance, you will be creating even more of a mineral deficit.

The main minerals to cleanse your blood are sodium, potassium, and magnesium. All are important and, as with everything else on your program, we need to make sure we have the correct balance of these items to boost your health.

Why Sodium (Salt) is Important

For decades, we've all been told that salt is bad for us and that we should cut it out of our diet. But as usual, this advice is misleading.

Blood sugar isn't affected by salt, but not getting enough salt can still affect our blood because without enough salt your circulating blood volume shrinks. Think about that for a second. With less salt in your body, your circulation is worse, and if it shrinks too much, you'll pass out. Salt depletion also means your body must compensate by using potassium from your kidneys just to retain more sodium. By losing potassium you run the risk of nausea, dehydration, frequent urination, sluggishness, and if things get too bad, confusion, paralysis and a messed-up heart rhythm.

On the other hand, eating less salt *is* important if (and only if) we are eating a lot of processed food because usually processed foods contain way more sodium than you need in a day. Doctors are right to tell people to limit the amount of sodium they eat if they eat poorly in the first place but ignoring it completely is unhelpful.

People with high blood pressure are often told to reduce salt by their doctors, but it's not because salt is bad for you. When you have high blood pressure coupled with a lot of salt in your food it can be a problem. This salt can lead to the body retaining more water and this additional fluid is pulled into the arteries and veins, which you want to avoid because that can raise your blood pressure even more. Hence, the need to reduce salt with high blood pressure.

You also need a good balance of salt in your diet if you are on an exercise regime, or if you're somebody who sweats a lot. This is because when we sweat, we also lose salt. Therefore, the combination for many of avoiding salt, plus exercising will mean your blood volume decreases, and that can lead to fatigue and can be potentially life-threatening if left unchecked.

One last thing to remember. When you reduce carbohydrates in your meals and continue to reduce sodium, you're going to feel lousy. You'll feel so tired and sluggish that you might conclude your lower carb diet isn't working because you feel so bad. However, it's not the diet, it's the amount of salt you *don't* have in your body, which again makes your potassium levels drop. By maintaining good salt and potassium levels you'll feel a lot better.

Why Potassium is Important

Having a good sodium to potassium balance is extremely important for healthy cell function, and if you've ever been told by your doctor that you have low potassium, the first thing they are going to recommend you add to your diet are bananas and orange juice. Both of which are terrible ideas for somebody with your condition because of the high sugar value of those two items.

Too often doctors can be outdated with their recommendations. Did you know there is as much potassium in 4oz of beef as there is in a medium banana or a glass of orange juice? Plus, there are zero carbs in meat which is ideal for helping reduce your blood sugar. You can eat a lot of avocado, spinach, or salmon to get a good amount of potassium – just avoid the bananas and juice.

Why Magnesium is Important

Our bones contain around 65% magnesium, and our muscles around 25%, with only about 1% in our bloodstream. This is why it can be hard to determine if you are deficient in magnesium through a blood test. Your test can still come back as normal and yet you can still be deficient in magnesium.[35]

Magnesium is important because it helps in the production of hormones (which you'll know if you read the **Your Blood** section), the production of energy, while also controlling the proper function of your muscles, namely their contraction and relaxation. This is ultra-important for the main muscle in the body, your heart. Overall, magnesium is a significant mineral.

When our magnesium levels are healthy, then our muscles are generally healthy but when our mineral levels are depleted the calming effect of magnesium is lost and the muscles begin to get a little twitchy, and by twitchy, I mean cramping – and that hurts.

If you regularly wake in the night with a cramp in your calf, that's a classic sign that you're low on magnesium. Severe magnesium depletion can also lead to your brain cramping, aka seizures. And if your heart cramps, well, that usually means death. I know that sounds extreme, but it also highlights the importance of magnesium.

Just like sodium and potassium, magnesium depletion can happen when we become dehydrated. However, it can also be caused by excessive sweating, sleep deprivation, or not eating enough food containing magnesium. The good news, just like the other minerals, is that this is easy to rectify.

There's a lot of magnesium in meat, which if you are a meat eater is great news. To make sure you get all the nutrients from your meat, make sure it's not processed meat, and make sure you don't boil or overcook your meat otherwise you'll lose all the nutrients from it. There's also a lot of magnesium in dark leafy greens, like spinach, chard and kale. As with meat, don't boil vegetables because you'll lose all the nutrients. Steam vegetables or eat them raw to ingest the highest amount of the minerals.

If you do experience cramps, you'll want to get rid of the problem quickly, and I always recommend a product called Nuun Electrolyte tablets, which are available from most grocery stores or online. These tablets contain electrolytes which include sodium, potassium, and magnesium. It can help to have one tablet a day until you finish the tube of ten tablets and your leg cramps should be gone. These tablets will tide you over until you are eating well enough that you are getting healthy amounts of magnesium from your food.

There are many other products that contain magnesium but stay away from Milk of Magnesia as this will pass through the body without much of the magnesium being absorbed. It can also lead to diarrhea which will again dehydrate you, potentially leading to more mineral loss.

Water is an Essential

The second essential Pillar in my list for optimal health is water, and it really is an essential that's often overlooked. Hydration is not only a terrific addition to losing weight, if that's another of your goals, but critical for your body to function well. If you remember, a human being is made up of around 60% water and more importantly, your brain and heart are made up of around 73% water. This means any form of dehydration, even the smallest amount, can affect you cognitively, emotionally and physically.

When I talk about dehydration, I don't mean the type of dehydration you might experience when lost in a desert for a day or two, I'm talking about being around 2% lower than optimal on the amount of water you might drink in a day. And realistically, most people I've worked with are way below 2% dehydrated in a day.

At the beginning of my client's journey, most drink very little water in a day. When I ask: "How much water do you drink in a day?" This is often the reply: "*I don't like water.*" Followed up with: "*I'll drink a glass of milk in the morning, have about three large cups of coffee during the day, with two or three sodas, and maybe some wine (or beer) in the evening."*

This is not drinking water. Yes, these are fluids but coffee and soda act as diuretics which mean they'll make you urinate and lose water. Milk is full of sugar, which we want to avoid; and alcohol dehydrates you, which will only compound the problem.

For years the Government recommendation of water intake is around eight glasses of 8oz a day. That total of 64oz, which is pretty good but in my opinion is still too low. If you're not drinking enough water in a day, one of the most usual signs of dehydration is feeling hungry, and the reason for this is that the body gets fluid from food. Hence your body will find a way to get some fluid it needs. But then this leads us to eat more and problems like diabetes, prediabetes and metabolic syndrome can follow. The cycle of poor health can start just from not drinking enough water.

Common Signs of Dehydration

- Foggy brain (cognitive impairment)
- Confusion
- Fatigue and sleepiness during the day
- Dry mouth
- Decreased urine flow
- Darker yellow to brown urine color
- Headaches
- Dizziness
- Blood pressure drop (can lead to fainting when you stand up quickly)
- Rapid heart rate
- Chest pains
- Seizure

Your goal should ideally to drink around 80 to 100oz of water a day. That's close to ten to twelve 8oz glasses of water, or up to three liters. Most of that volume should come from plain water, but you can also use herbal tea, broth, and naturally flavored sparkling water.

Strategies for Drinking More Water

If you are a person who doesn't drink much water or doesn't like drinking plain water, then here are my tips to help you get to 100oz of water in a day.

The Nike Solution

If I may borrow a slogan from Nike, *Just do it*! Many people with your condition don't like plain water because they're so used to drinking sweet drinks, like soda. In the beginning, water might seem plain and lacking flavor, but once you are able to drop a lot of the sweet foods and drinks from your diet, then your taste buds will change, and you'll be able to taste subtle flavors - and water is subtle. You'll also find the more you drink, the more you get used to it. The more you get used to it, the more you'll notice when you're not drinking enough.

Go Big or Go Home

Get a large bottle, maybe a liter size (or bigger) bottle or mug and keep it with you the entire day. Sip regularly from it. Don't wait until you're thirsty, just keep sipping. The problem with drinking a lot in one go is you can feel very full, and even nauseous. But taking a sip every few minutes the task of drinking more is a lot easier, and soon you get into the habit of topping yourself up regularly. After years of drinking about 100oz a day, I really notice if I don't drink enough. Because of that I have a large cup with me during the day - a 50oz Reduce vacuumed-insulated tumbler (www.reduceeveryday.com) which I love because it makes it easy to keep track of how much I drink. If I drink two full cups, then I've hit my 100oz for the day. This is a lot easier than filling a small cup or bottle multiple times a day.

Get a Straw

This may sound weird, but once you have your bottle or large cup with you, then try and make sure you sip your water from a straw. For some reason, drinking from a straw makes drinking water easier, which is another reason why I love my Reduce tumbler (and no, they don't sponsor me... but I am available!). Maybe it's some type of throwback to when I was a young child drinking a milkshake, or maybe as a baby having to suck milk from my mother or a bottle? Whatever the reason, drinking with a straw can be a valuable for increasing your water intake.

Set an Alarm

If you keep forgetting to drink, set an alarm on your phone to remind you to make sure you've had around 10oz every hour during the day. If you do this from 9 am to around 7 pm, you'll get your 100oz per day.

Track Your Progress

Some people find it helpful to track their water on an app. There are several options out there and one I like is called *Daily Water: Drink Tracker and Reminder*. With this app, you can set a water goal and a schedule for when to drink. It will then remind you when to drink. Very helpful if you like to gamify your goals.

Fill Up Early

When you first wake up, you're dehydrated from not drinking for 8 hours. The first thing you can do before you even get out of bed is have your bottle or cup next to your bed and drink down as much as you can. If you can drink close to 20oz before you even get up, you're one-fifth of the way to your daily goal. The good news with drinking so much early is you are probably going to need to urinate anyway, so drinking more water at this point isn't going to inconvenience you.

Make Spa Water

If you find plain water a little dull, then making spa water might be the way to go. Spa water is basically water with added fruit or vegetables in it to give it a light, natural flavor. My favorite spa water mix is to add cucumber and raspberries together into a bottle of water and let it infuse during the day. Once you've finished the water, just refill and you'll continue to have flavored water. You can use other produce like oranges, strawberries, ginger, cinnamon, apples, peaches or kiwi fruit for a fun variety

The best way to prepare your spa water is to cut your fruit or vegetable into thin slices and load them into your bottle. To keep most of the flavor in the water, once you get to around a 1/3 of water left in your bottle or cup, go refill and continue drinking.

Don't Go Cold

Apart from drinking iced water in the summer, drinking icy water the rest of the year isn't always the easiest thing to do. In the cooler months, I find keeping my water at room temperature makes it easier to drink. And in the winter months, when it can be a lot harder to drink icy water, I recommend drinking warm or hot water. This can still be plain water, but you can use caffeine-free herbal tea for a more interesting, soothing drinking experience. Hot water in the winter is a lot easier to get down than cold.

Sip by Sip

If you're not used to drinking a lot of water in a day, it can be hard to go from a little to a lot overnight. I recommend that you build up slowly towards 100oz over a few weeks. Work on drinking at least 60oz of water in a day, and then add 10oz a week for the next month. By then you should find getting close to 100oz is achievable. Like all things mentioned in this book, take everything at a pace that feels comfortable to you and know that even the smallest steps mean you're making progress.

Notes on Drinking More Water

In the beginning, drinking more water and eating well is going to make you go to the bathroom more often. The first couple of weeks you might find you are urinating a lot; and by a lot, I mean every 30 minutes or less. This is a good sign, and one that means your body is starting to hydrate, which sounds a little backward. When we're dehydrated, we don't urinate as much, as when we are hydrated. Which is why, as your body adjusts, you'll go from peeing a few times a day to a few times an hour. After a couple of weeks, you'll find your able to drink more water without urinating as much as your body starts to find a comfortable balance.

Pillar #3: Nutrition

Most people on a new health program usually start off by prioritizing food as the area to change the most, and although I feel sleep and water are more important to balance first, the fact that we eat multiple time a day does make the nutrition Pillar a common starting point.

In fact, you'll probably spend more time in the Nutrition section than anywhere else in this book. But before you get there, let's understand what we mean by nutrition and how it influences your condition. I'll talk more about how nutrition affects your body in the **Blood Work** section, but here's a quick breakdown.

Protein

When you think of eating protein, you might have thoughts of bodybuilders eating massive amounts of chicken to create bigger muscles. That is something they do, however, building muscle is only one function of protein. And there are many other significant reasons to make sure protein is your priority macro-nutrient. These are the types of nutrients the body needs in large amounts. In this book macro-nutrients refer to protein, fats and carbohydrates.

Protein is the building block to the function and structure of every living cell in your body, and it's surprisingly a macro-nutrient many people under-eat. In the nutrition section I'll cover more about protein options and quantities but here are a few points of information you might find interesting:

The etymology of protein is from the Greek word 'primary', which is why protein should be the first macro-nutrient to focus on when changing any diet choices. Protein is found in both animal and plant protein, yet animal protein is closer to our human amino makeup than plants, but both can be used to fulfill your daily protein needs. Unfortunately, just having plant protein will typically involve eating a whole lot more food, which isn't always convenient.

What makes protein so good as a dietary source is our body absorbs protein efficiently, which means we have less waste because it's absorbed. Unlike carbohydrates, which we know are often left floating around our blood in the form of glucose.

Protein is found in our muscle as well as other structural components like skin, blood, myosin and actin (both form muscle cells), collagen (the most abundant protein found in the body) and hemoglobin (a molecule which carries oxygen from the lungs around the body, and carbon dioxide back to the lungs).

There are twenty common amino acids found in protein, and nine of these are classed as *essential* to the human body. These nine amino acids cannot be created by the body, so it is *essential* that we get them from food sources. Animal proteins contain all nine essential amino acids and are called 'complete' proteins. Plant proteins (except soybeans) on the other hand are lacking in one or more of the essential amino acids and are therefore called 'incomplete' proteins.

The Nine Essential Amino Acids We Get From Food

- Histidine
- Isoleucine
- Leucine
- Lysine
- Methionine
- Phenylalanine
- Threonine
- Tryptophan
- Valine

How Much Protein is Enough?

It is true that you can eat too much protein. The body is only able to store a small percentage of protein, and then the extra amino acids are turned into glucose, which is something we want to avoid if we want to cleanse our blood.

The Recommended Dietary Allowance (RDA) of protein coming from the U.S. Department of Agriculture (USDA) is rather too low in my humble opinion. The USDA recommends a person eats around 0.4g of protein per pound of bodyweight. But you need to bear in mind the USDA is recommending a minimum amount of protein which should be eaten by an average sized person in a day, and not the optimum amount if you are to be healthy.

To function at a high level, especially if you plan to reverse your condition, lose weight, exercise, or a combination of all three, then you would clearly need more protein than this recommendation.

Most nutrition rating systems have traditionally been based on recommended calories in a day (I'll explain why this is a bad idea in depth at the end of this section) but this focus on calories is next to meaningless for healthy, balanced eating. The truth is, it's not about how many calories we eat in a day that matters, but where those calories come from. It's essential we have a good balance of proteins, fats, and carbohydrates, and *when* we eat them that makes a difference to our health.

I much prefer that we move away from the idea of calorie counting. Rather we should make sure we eat the right amount of food for each meal and at the right time. This combination is going to offer the most realistic way to give you enough fuel while balancing your blood sugar.[37, 38]

My recommendation for the amount of protein to eat a day would be closer to 0.75g of protein per pound of body weight for adults under 64 years of age. And if you are above 64 years old, research shows us that older people require even more protein than young adults for healthy body maintenance. This is mainly due to the fact protein deficiency affects all organs, including the heart, brain and the immune system. As we get older, we need to maintain healthy organs, which is why protein again is so important. For those of you 64 and up, to maintain healthy muscle mass and bone density, I'd go with 1g-1.2g of protein per body pound of weight as the ideal.[36]

As you can see, this is far different from the generalize 0.4g from the USDA. At the end of the day, it is you who makes the decision on how much protein to eat, I just recommend that you make it your priority food option to cleanse your blood.

Fats

Fat in all its guises - saturated, monounsaturated and polyunsaturated - has been much maligned for over 50+ years. For far too long, people have been told to avoid fat if they want to avoid heart disease and be healthy. Well, like most things when it comes to food and health, the advice is confusing and often still based on debunked science.

A mix of healthy fats is essential for overall good health and weight maintenance. In fact, there is no association between dietary saturated fat and an increase in cardiovascular disease or diabetes.[39,40,41,42] You didn't misread that -- there is *no* relevant evidence that saturated or other healthy fats increase your risk of heart disease or diabetes.

Another reason fat was targeted as the item to be removed from food is because of the ridiculous calorie counting fad that has really done more harm than good. If you are trying to reduce your calories, the easiest way to do that is remove all fat from your diet and that's because each gram of fat contains 9 calories. If you compare that with 4 calories for protein and 4 calories for carbohydrates, you can see why removing the higher number food gives you better numbers.

But numbers are not what keep people healthy. By removing fat from processed and packaged foods, manufacturers could claim the benefit of their low-calorie product, appeasing people who bought into fad claims and dangerously unhelpful guidelines.

This, for me, is the main reason why there is a diabetes and obesity epidemics in the USA and around the world. Removing fat and increasing quick processed carbs like pasta into our overly saturated carb focused meals has put more people at risk of health problems.

When I explain the importance of fats to my clients, I often get the same unsure look I'm imagining you have on your face right now, and maybe the same comment: *"It's hard to embrace fats after being told to avoid them for so long."* This is a valid comment and I understand it.

But let's talk about this in relation to our hormone leptin. If we don't eat enough fats in our diet, we are not going to be physically satisfied. If we're not satisfied our leptin levels are going to stay high and high leptin levels means you want to eat more food (I explain in **Your Blood** why balancing our hormones is). Fats not only control your hunger cravings but also help you feel more satiated. The more satisfied you are, the easier it is to eat healthy portions. Plus, food will also taste better with fats in it. And very importantly, fats will give your body more energy as it's a slower burning energy than carbohydrates.

Now you know, fat is your friend.

Carbohydrates

Carbs come in many guises which can be a little confusing because not all carbs are equal in the benefits we gain from them. However, all carbs become glucose in our blood once they've been processed by our digestive system. This is why we need to be mindful that a carb is a carb is a carb, no matter where it comes from.

However, carbs are not all evil. There are two types of carbohydrates: Simple and Complex. Simple carbs tend to break down quickly in our gut and get absorbed into our blood very fast. This is the type of carb that spikes our blood sugar creating a large insulin release and this is bad for you and your blood condition.

Then we have Complex carbs. These carbs breakdown slower, mainly because they are fibrous. However, the Complex carbs in something like an apple still become glucose in your body, just the same as the Simple carbs in a chocolate bar. It just does it more slowly than the Simple carb. Either way, with your blood condition, these carbs still need to be cleansed from your blood.

I'll show you what your best carbohydrate options are in the Nutrition section, but a general rule of thumb - Complex is better than Simple.

Simple Carbs

These carbs are quickly and easily broken down into glucose almost immediately after eating. These carbs simply offer no nutritional value to you and really should be avoided completely.

- All sugars (white or brown)
- All syrups (corn, maple etc.)
- Jams
- Fruit drinks
- Soda
- Candy

Pretty much anything that's unnaturally sweet will be a Simple carb. Part of the problem we face these days is that carbohydrates are in so much of what we eat, even in food where they don't belong. Take beef jerky as an example. If you look at the label on a beef jerky packet, typically the second ingredient is brown sugar! Seriously.

Simple carbs are the carbohydrates you do need to avoid if you want to lower and manage your blood sugar.

Complex Carbs

The second type of carbohydrate is a Complex carb. These carbs are a little different because they tend to contain fiber and vitamins which do contain some nutritional value for us.
- Fruit
- Vegetables
- Legumes (beans, lentils, chickpeas etc.)
- Nuts

What makes these carbs more important is the fiber they contain. Even though too many Complex carbs are still not healthy for us. The slower the absorption, the less of a blood sugar spike we experience, which means less insulin released into our blood.

Carbs are Non-Essential

Apart from both types of carbs turning to glucose in your body, they share another commonality, they are *non-essential* macro-nutrients. Unlike protein which contains *essential* amino acids which our body does need for health, carbohydrates are not essential for any function in the body. This is because if the body is deficient in carbohydrates it will turn protein into glucose, and voila! you have the glucose needed for healthy functioning.

The truth is you can survive without any carbs, but that wouldn't be something I'd not recommend just because life would be boring without them. Also, your brain does appreciate having a minimal amount of carbs to help it work.

Net Carb Nonsense

Now you know the difference between Simple and Complex carbs, and how they are absorbed into the blood, let me warn you about the new trend in food manufacturing called Net Carbs (also known as impact carbs).

The theory behind Net Carbs is that if you subtract the amount of fiber a food has from your carbohydrate total, then that fiber will somehow negate those carbs. Many low-carb companies have been using Net Carbs on a lot of processed foods to try to convince people into thinking the carb content of their products are lower than they are, therefore making their foods more appealing. But the truth is Net Carbs are not a real thing, and you won't find them on the legal Nutrition Fact label. And that's because this theory isn't approved by the Federal Drug Agency (FDA) whose job it is to ensure the safety of food products.

So, how do these companies get away with putting Net Carbs on the packet when the theory isn't conclusively backed by research? Because they are sneaky and clever. You can claim anything on the packaging of a food product as long as what is on the Nutrition Facts label is true. Essentially, a company could call the same 'theory' *Unicorn Carbs*, and it would mean the same thing - nothing.

If we think about this Net Carbs claim, then we could think of all Complex carbs (apple, nuts etc.) in the same way because they all contain fiber. Alas, this is not true. Even though fiber does slow down the absorption of carbs in the gut, it doesn't remove the glucose that's entering your bloodstream. It's true you will get less of a spike of insulin released but you'll still get insulin. And if you are insulin resistant, which you most probably are with diabetes, prediabetes or metabolic syndrome, then this glucose is still a problem in your blood.

A lot of these Net Carb products also contain sugar-alcohols. These sugar alcohols tend to be sugar-free, which also lower the calorie count, but still keep the food tasting sweet. They have names like

Xylitol, Erythritol or Sorbitol. But be careful with Net Carbs and food containing sugar-alcohols because research is clear that food sweetened with sugar-alcohols still have the same impact on blood glucose.[43]

Think about this. If the Net Carbs theory were true, all I'd need to do is eat a couple of donuts and down a glass of Metamucil fiber drink to negate the carbs. Do you really think that would help reverse your blood condition?

Don't be fooled, research on Net Carbs is very fuzzy and not at all conclusive and as we can't trust food manufacturers to have your best interests at heart. I say ignore these unfounded claims if you want to get healthy.

Why Calorie Counting is a Bad Idea

I've mentioned calorie counting is a bad idea, so I wanted to give you my take on this subject and you can make up your own mind.

If you've ever tried to lose weight in the past, I bet you've heard this widely-held belief a million times: *'If you eat more calories than you burn, you'll get fat. And the easiest way to lose weight is to eat fewer calories and exercise more because you burn off more calories.'*

But I'm here to tell you, this is wrong, wrong, wrong and wrong again. The trouble is, we've been bombarded with this nonsense for the best part of 40 years and the latest health fad of counting steps and knowing how many calories you've burned, does not help. The reality is reversing your blood condition, losing weight and getting healthy comes down to what we eat and how often we eat; it is not about how many calories we eat.

To give you a simple example of why counting calories isn't a helpful way of gauging which foods to eat, we'll examine a so-called healthy food option.

Fruit Smoothie Example

Nutrition Facts

1 servings per container

Serving size	1 (1g)

Amount Per Serving

Calories 230

	% Daily Value*
Total Fat 0g	0%
Saturated Fat 0g	0%
Trans Fat 0g	
Sodium 10mg	0%
Total Carbohydrate 57g	21%
Dietary Fiber 2g	7%
Total Sugars 47g	
Includes 0g Added Sugars	0%
Protein 1g	2%

Not a significant source of cholesterol, vitamin D, calcium, iron, and potassium

*The % Daily Value (DV) tells you how much a nutrient in a serving of food contributes to a daily diet. 2,000 calories a day is used for general nutrition advice.

Over the last 10 years, smoothies and juicing has become the nutrition fad to get you into shape. The idea is that you can drink a healthy fruit or vegetable drink, that is relatively low in calories, instead of eating food will help you lose weight and be healthy. Sounds great? Well, let's have a look at the label of a well-known smoothie drink bottle to see the truth.

Most processed food packages and bottles will have some type of reference to being low calorie on the front. And this smoothie manufacturer is no different. This strawberry and banana smoothie label claims to contain only 230 calories, which sounds great. But wait, let's look at what's really going on inside this bottle by examining the label. If you're not up to speed on reading labels, I recommend you go to the **Food Label** chapter in the **Nutrition** section.

230 calories seems quite reasonable but have a look at how many carbohydrates are in this bottle: 57g grams. That is astronomical! And of that 47g is sugar alone.

Think about this. If there are 4g of carbohydrates in a single sugar cube, this smoothie drink has the equivalent of 14 sugar cubes in it. Would you really want to drink 14 sugar cubes? This smoothie also contains only 2g of fiber, therefore we know these carbs are going to be absorbed into the body very quickly. And fast carbs equal a big insulin release, something you need to avoid. This smoothie also contains zero fat, which means this won't fill you up. But if we are only counting calories, then none of that should matter, right?

Do you know what else contains 230 calories and is really good for you? A chicken breast. That same chicken breast also contains zero carbs.

If we take calorie counting as the best way to estimate how much food we should eat or not eat, then the theory is claiming a smoothie drink with the equivalent of 14 sugar cubes has the same nutritional value as a chicken breast with zero sugar in it? I don't know about you, but that example alone makes calorie counting seem idiotic.

The other part of the above flawed statement of calorie counters is 'you need to burn more calories than you eat' to be thin and healthy. Really? Let's look at this. Calories in, Calories out (CICO) is based on the theory garnered from the laws of thermodynamics. And specifically, the first law of thermodynamics which is called a 'conservation law'. This law states that the form of energy may change, which in our case is protein, carbs or fat, but the total is always conserved (all calories are the same). Seems perfectly simple, right? You eat 1700 calories, then those 1700 calories are turned to energy in your body, no more, and no less. So, in theory, if you stick to a reduced calorie-controlled diet, eat fewer calories while burning more calories than you eat, just like magic, you'll lose weight and be healthy. Well, no, it's not that simple.

If we look at the comparable calories of the juice drink to a chicken breast – and I'm sure by now you can clearly understand there's a nutritional difference between the two, especially on how it impacts your blood sugar. But what the CICO theory suggests is that these two items act the same way in the body because it's just about calories. But they don't work the same in the body. And they don't have the same function in the body. Remember, protein is essential for your body function, carbohydrates are not. This makes CICO an unhelpful approach because the theory overlooks the biological and hormonal responses to the food we eat. If you eat all 1700 calories from sugar, that is going to have a very different effect on you and your blood than eating 1700 from protein and fat.

Another reason CICO is inaccurate is that our system has a third option other than simply calories in and calories out, and that's called 'fat storage'. Nearly all calories coming into our body are turned into glucose energy. Some of this energy is expelled through how our body heals itself, through our vital organs or muscle usage (basal metabolism) but we're still going to be left with a lot of glucose energy in our system if we've eaten excess carbohydrates, and we know this extra glucose will have to be stored away as fat. You can't out exercise excessive glucose in your blood.

Therefore, those 'calories in' do not just go straight out or get burned, but *stay in*. The decision on how these calories are used has nothing to do with calories but where those calories come from, and how much glucose is produced from those calories.

Bread and sugar raise insulin levels, therefore more calories from these sources are going to lead to more insulin release and more fat storage than if we ate something like butter or cheese. This theory of CICO doesn't address the important topics of insulin release or insulin sensitivity.

But here's the kicker. To lose one pound of body fat, you need to shed around 3,500 calories. For a 180-pound person, an hour's workout tends to burn around 150-300 calories.[95]

That smoothie is 230 calories. Do you know what's easier and better for you than working out for that hour and counting calories? Don't drink the smoothie and you've done better for your blood health by avoiding that ridiculous amount of sugar.

Counting calories and exercising to burn those calories just doesn't make sense, when you can make better choices to cleanse your blood. Sleep better, drink more, eat healthy, reduce your stress and then exercise for fun. Do that first and you'll be doing a whole lot more for yourself than obsessively counting calories and driving yourself mad.

Pillar #4: Stress

Stress is one of the more difficult Pillars to quantify because it tends to be a catch-all word for something that affects us physically, behaviorally, cognitively, emotionally and hormonally. Whatever we decide to call stress, the effects of it can have major implications for our overall health and wellbeing. Although I rank stress as an important Pillar to balance but not essential, that doesn't mean we shouldn't pay attention to it.

It's fair to say we all have certain levels of stress in our life. Some can be short-term, and others chronic but no matter what your stress level is, it will have an impact on your blood condition and high and prolonged stress will only make your condition worse.

I think we're all familiar with the term 'stress' but in truth, stress can mean anything from being anxious, fearful, worried, bored, overwhelmed, frustrated or even sick. Stress is often a generalization used to describe any situation where we have a negative feeling about ourselves, others or the world. But whatever your experience, or meaning, stress will impact our mental, physical, emotional and behavioral wellbeing in the same ways, because when we feel stressed our body believes it's under attack.

Our response to this attack is where the term fight or flight comes from. However, there is also another response not regularly mentioned, the freeze response. All three of these responses are known as the acute stress response, where the body reacts when faced with an anxiety-provoking experience.

Almost all your body systems - the heart, lungs, sensory organs, the brain, immune system and blood vessels - are affected when one of these responses is triggered. In cases of actual threat, this can be extremely important. Imagine you're out on a hike and you come across a grizzly bear. Within seconds your brain has acknowledged the real threat and without conscious thought, your acute stress response kicks in and you do one of three things: run away; freeze on the spot with the hope it walks off; or you act aggressively to scare it off. This is our system working perfectly. But what happens in modern life when we don't have those obvious threats?

Well, something else can trigger these responses and that is when we perceive a threat, any threat. The trouble with this type of anxiety thinking is in our modern society even the smallest problem in our imagination can lead to the greatest threat to our survival. But how does this happen?

Let me give you a common example from past clients:

Fred is hard working. He goes to work every day and does the best he can. He has a family with three daughters. He loves them all and would do anything for them. One day, Fred finds out that his boss isn't happy with a job he did. Fred begins to worry that he might lose his job, so he starts working harder to rectify his mistake. He begins to work longer hours. Every job he starts he fears getting it wrong because he doesn't want to lose his job.

Fred begins showing signs of anxiety. He imagines that if he loses his job, he won't be able to feed his family. He starts imagining his wife leaving him and taking the children because he can't provide. He imagines losing the house and having nowhere to live. He imagines living rough on the street. He imagines drinking himself to death under a bridge. These thoughts become common to Fred and in time, any hint in his life that he has done something wrong, he automatically goes from being okay, to being dead under a bridge in under five seconds.

What this thinking does is begin to trigger his acute stress responses earlier and earlier. This happens because the more he imagines these terrible things happening, the more his brain believe it to be true. His brain actually believes this threat is real! Fred has gone from an imagined threat to himself and his family, to believing this is an actual threat to his life.

This might sound extreme, but it really isn't. I've heard this story countless times from people who have become very sick because stress in their life has turned into a chronic problem. This is why for some people even getting an email from their boss can send them into a panic. They may not know why, because their acute stress response has kicked in, but somewhere in their mind a real threat to their survival has been triggered.

What is relevant to your condition, is that it doesn't matter which of these responses you face, or the severity of your response, the same thing is happening in your body. An important hormone called Cortisol is being dumped into your blood stream.

Cortisol primes your body for action by making more glucose available to your muscles for you to run or fight if need be. The problem comes when you have diabetes, prediabetes or metabolic syndrome and have become what is known as *insulin resistant*. Because you have high blood sugar anyway, the extra glucose that gets dumped into your bloodstream is going to make it even higher. And this makes you sicker.

Our fight, flight or freeze response is only supposed to be a short-term response to an acute threat but in our modern society, we tend to be under stress for longer periods, which means our acute stress response could be broken just like Fred's.

Over time, this long-term Cortisol release causes havoc with your blood, which can be one reason why you may have the condition you have even if everything else in your life is quite healthy. Your blood condition might be due to the amount of stress you're under every single day.

Strategies for Reducing Stress

As I noted before, stress and anxiety are close bed-fellows and it's beyond the scope of this book to go into how to understand and manage chronic anxiety in any significant way. However, there are a few things I recommend you can do to help minimize the stress most of us experience daily. Now, I say minimize because the reality is you might not be able to change much about the environmental or workload stresses you're under. But what you can learn to do is not let these everyday stresses overwhelm you and create the internal impact we all know has a detrimental effect on your blood sugar and insulin levels.

The 30/60 Rule

This is essentially making sure that for every 30 minutes you are inactive or sedentary, you get up and do 60 seconds of activity. The intensity of this activity is up to you. You might want to walk for 60 seconds or you might want to sprint on the spot or do jumping jacks for 60 seconds. Even walking to the bathroom counts. It doesn't really matter what you do, as long as you do something. We do this 30/60 because physical inactivity is associated with the development of insulin resistance and increased blood pressure, both of which we know isn't good for reversing your condition.[89,90]

If you're stuck in the car or a long meeting that goes on longer than 30 minutes, then make sure for every 30 minutes you didn't move you make up for it at the end. So, if you were in a meeting for two hours, at the end of that meeting you make sure you move around for two minutes, it's that simple.

This 30/60 rule isn't about exercise but about moving your body to help reduce cortisol (stress hormone) and to reduce insulin resistance. If you can incorporate this into your daily activity, you'll be making substantial changes to your stress levels with little effort.

Keep a Journal

Yeah, I know, this sounds like something out of a Jane Austen novel, but the reality is that writing down your thoughts and how you feel about certain situations can really help to reduce stress and blood pressure while increasing critical thinking.[91,92] Being able to move your thoughts from your head to something outside of yourself can really help with gaining perspective on problems you may face.

The reason for this is if we think about something over and over, our brain will assume it's important and it will create more thinking space to accommodate the thoughts. This often means other things get pushed to the background, and before we know it, we start to focus almost entirely on the problem we're anxious about. You've probably noticed this when something is on your mind, and it ends up being the only thing you can think about.

And because we are constantly thinking about this stressor, our body begins to experience all the physical and emotional symptoms that accompany stress, which then amplifies the problem. Our brain interprets these stress feelings and sensations as an attack on our safety and wellbeing and it starts to focus entirely on the problem to find a solution, even if there isn't a solution. In time, by ruminating on a problem we get caught in a spiraling pattern that is hard to get out of. And to top it off, our cortisol release is rising and rising pushing our blood sugar, insulin levels, and blood pressure through the roof. All this from just from thinking about a problem!

Therefore, I say keep a journal. It's the simplest way to combat any ruminating. I recommend you take about 20 minutes a week (or even a day if your anxiety thinking is that pervasive) to jot down any stressful thoughts you have. Just as I did in the sleep section, I highly recommended writing down thoughts before bed to aid sleep. This might include conversations you had with people and how you felt about what was said or not said. Sometimes writing down what we wanted to do and say has some power in freeing us from ruminating on our 'failings' in a situation.

Write down your concerns about the issue contributing to your stress. Have a dialogue with yourself because this back-and-forth can sometimes help you to find a solution to problems you might not have thought about.

You might also want to try an exercise of write down a continuous stream-of-thought. This is writing without thinking. You write and don't stop, you just write and let your mind wander. This can be a very creative experience and leads to hidden thoughts which you might have been avoiding or not aware of.

The idea behind stream-of-thought writing is not to care about the content, spelling or grammar, just write and let anything which is bouncing around your head come out.

I'm often asked if electronic journaling is as effective as old-fashioned writing on paper. I find if you have specific stresses and problems which could do with a solution, then writing on paper seems to be more beneficial. However, if you're just writing a stream of thought to get thoughts out of your head, then typing can be a lot faster.

Whatever way you choose to do it, just give it a try.

Meditate Daily

Okay, be honest, what was your first reaction to this tip? Many people I recommend meditation to just shake their heads and dismiss it straight away. But I've got to tell you, this is one of the best ways to deal with everyday stress. I think meditation has had such a bad rap for so long, with people thinking it's cultish, or for hippies and yogis but not everyday people.

Meditation doesn't need to take hours to be effective. You can meditate from anywhere between 5 to 30 minutes a day to experience some meaningful changes in your thinking. What mediation does is give your brain a mini-vacation from your stress. You may have tried to meditate before but found it hard to do and didn't get back to it. This often happens because people think meditating means they have to have a mind empty of thoughts and get annoyed when they can't achieve this state. But this isn't true. Maybe highly-experienced monks can do that but for the rest of us, intrusive thoughts will pop in and out.

What we can learn to do with meditation is to let thoughts pass by like birds in the sky. We can learn to notice them and let them fly on. It's a great way to learn not to dwell on thoughts.

Whether you're new to meditation or have participated in the activity for a while, I still recommend you get a meditation buddy, and for this, I use either the Mindspace app (mindspace.com) or the Calm app (calm.com). I think both are excellent for introducing people to the benefits of meditation in a slow, fun and effective way.

If you don't like the idea of meditating, then think of it as a deep breathing exercise to calm the mind; because it's basically the same thing.

Quiet Time

Along with meditation, I think it is becoming increasingly important to have quiet time during the day, even if you don't want to meditate. These days we are always connected to something, whether it's our smartphone, email or TV. There's always some electronic gadget or technology we're plugged into and I think this is having a detrimental effect on our inner world. And this, in turn, causes more stress.

We've only had the Internet and smartphones for the past 30 years but already they are taking over our lives. You've probably observed people who are waiting in a doctor's office or the checkout line, and the first thing they do rather than stand and wait is pull out their smartphone and start looking at something. It's like people are forgetting how to be quiet or just be with our own mind for company.

It's like if we're not being entertained every second of the day, then we're missing something.

Let me ask you this: *"When was the last time you went out for the day and left your smartphone at home? And, if it wasn't on purpose, how did you feel without it?"* I think it's fair to say most people will get anxious if their phone isn't in their pocket - it's become like an electronic life preserver.

I'd like to encourage you to put time aside every day to cultivate a habit of being quiet. For at least 10 minutes a day, I'd like you to switch off your phone, your TV, and your computer, and just sit in silence not doing anything. Even though we may not be able to return to a world without invasive technology, taking time to unplug and be with ourselves can be a very useful way of finding ourselves again.

Get Outside

If you're cooped up in your office, car or house for an extended period, then I recommend getting outside for some fresh air. Ideally, I recommend going somewhere in nature like a forest or by water, although I know that isn't always possible. However, the act of moving to an outside space can help reduce stress, because the old saying by Winston Churchill is very true: 'A change is as good as a rest.'

Also, just like meditation, the idea of going outside is to encourage you to breathe and shake off any stress you might be carrying. This activity only needs to be for a few minutes but that few minutes can make an enormous difference.

If possible, take 10 to 15 minutes every day. And if you can do this while walking, you'll also be helping make your body more insulin sensitive which is great for helping reverse your condition.[93]

Socialize and Talk

A lot of people don't like to share how they feel about the stress they're under but socializing and talking to others is a very powerful tool against stress. Spending time with people who care and love you can offer equilibrium to your life by enforcing a sense of belonging, purpose, and fun, which counters the effects of stress and being locked into your internal thoughts. Being able to laugh with others, talk about your day, share a meal, or watch a movie with somebody can be a great stress reliever.

Now, if a friend or significant others is part of your stressor then you might want to talk to a therapist: *"But I'm not crazy,"* I hear you say. Well, a common misconception people have about talking to a therapist is they think they need to be depressed or have a mental health issue to do so, but that's just not true. Many therapists are happy to help you work through any problem or stressor you have which you feel might be bogging you down, no matter what that is.

As a psychotherapist, I'm happy to talk through thoughts and issues big or small. You don't have to be going through something huge like a divorce or job change for your stressor to be significant. Even something like: *"How do I tell my colleagues that I can't keep helping them with their projects?"* can be something to talk about.

Just like journaling, anything you can do to take thoughts out of your head helps give you some space from the internal chatter that can lead to increased stress.

Make a Change

Too often people will keep themselves in a stressful situation far too long before they do something about it. I've worked with so many people who are depressed because they've gone down this route, and I can tell you, being depressed or anxious while managing diabetes, prediabetes or metabolic syndrome is unlikely to feel easy. Sometimes we just need to accept that some situations and events which affect us aren't going to change, and to facilitate a healthy future for ourselves we just need to move on.

Making a change like leaving a job or a marriage is typically the last resort to reducing or eliminating stress. Often the thought of moving on from a stressful situation can compound our stress, even though we know instinctively it's the right thing to do. Too often I talk to people who stay in jobs or relationships because they're either afraid to move on, or the money they make is such that they are reluctant to lose what they have. But it always comes down to this one question. How much is your health and wellbeing worth to you? Because at the end of the day, your blood condition really is a potential killer and it doesn't matter what your job title is, or how much money you earn, if you're not around to enjoy your life.

Moving on and making big lifestyle changes can be a significant challenge, which is why the other tips in this list are usually the first to undertake to help reduce any stressors you have. However, if they don't help then it might be time to realize that if *you* can't change, and the situation isn't going to change, then the environment needs to change.

If you feel like you are stuck in this type of situation, I fully encourage you to seek out a therapist or life coach to talk through all the options before you, because talking with an unbiased third party, really can help you sort your thoughts out and move forward.

Pillar #5: Exercise

Exercise is often one of the first things recommended for lifestyle change, and many people believe their lack of exercise is why they have their blood condition. However, the trouble is, as I've mentioned before, exercising to reverse your condition and attain long-term weight loss isn't very effective at all.[30,44,45]

There are multiple issues with focusing on exercise as the primary way to get healthy, but these are often ignored by health professionals and the media. Most of my clients report that they've just been told to start exercising by their doctor and they have no clue as to what is effective, so they often end up doing the traditional exercises that magazines and media push as being 'the way' to get healthy. These include weight training, running or walking and counting steps. But the reality is that while exercises may be useful to some people, it's not that effective in reversing your blood condition.

The focus for exercise should be on doing what helps increase insulin sensitivity, and forgetting about anything else, including weight loss as your primary goal.[46,47] The reason for this is by increasing your insulin sensitivity, your body will be able to absorb more of the excess blood sugar, which will help your hormone system rebalance. And once you start to get your insulin and other hormones back in balance, then your triglycerides, blood pressure and any excess body fat will start to come down too. This is the key to getting healthy. It's not about how far you can run or walk or how much you can lift in the gym, it's how well balanced your hormones are, especially insulin.

If you do need to lose weight, you'll find increasing insulin sensitivity allows the body to release visceral adipose tissue, which is the fat around the abdominal cavity and organs. Focusing on fat loss over insulin sensitivity is really the wrong way to look at weight loss and reversing your condition. At the end of the day, it nearly always comes down to insulin sensitivity. Fixing that, will go a long way in fixing everything else.

If you read magazines or listen to many fitness instructors, you'll hear them say that exercise increases endorphins (the so-called 'feel-good' hormones), which is why you might feel good after exercise. Actually, there's little evidence to support this claim. However, what exercise is excellent for is reducing stress because exercise increases the concentration of *norepinephrine* in the brain. This is significant because fifty percent of norepinephrine is produced in a section of the brain called the *locus coeruleus*, which is the section of the brain involved in stress and emotional responses. The more norepinephrine the brain can produce, the more capable the brain is at responding to stress. This makes exercise a good addition to all the other Pillars, just don't put it at the top of your list.

Let's define what exercise means regarding cleansing your blood. Basically, it means 'any type of physical movement that significantly raises your heart rate above your normal resting heart rate for more than 10-15 minutes at least 3 times a week'.

The key part of this statement is that your exercise *raises* your heart rate. Time is not so important, as that is something to work towards. With increased heart rate as our goal, the right type of exercise for you is called High Intensity Interval training or HIIT.

Don't be put off by the name, HIIT is the most effective form of exercise over other forms of exercise because of its ability to raise and lower your heart rate in a short amount of time. It's this raising and lowering that makes HIIT so important and evidence supports HIIT as having a positive impact on glucose uptake in the muscles. That means HIIT is a terrific way to reverse insulin resistance and become more insulin sensitive, which is our main goal with doing exercise.[50, 51]

What happens during this HIIT process that works so well to cleanse your blood is this process of raising and lowering your heart rate. This up and down effect increases the citric acid cycle (Krebs cycle) in the liver. This essentially means your fuel molecules (glucose, fatty acids, and amino acids) are burnt off as energy in the liver. Because your condition means your blood sugar is typically high, what makes HIIT so good is directly helpful for reducing sugar in your blood, enabling fat loss and increased oxidization of this blood, thus lowering blood pressure. How good is that (fantastic if you didn't know)?

But what about ordinary resistance training you ask? Well, this can be good for increasing muscle mass and bone density and in time, resistance work is going to benefit you tremendously. But nothing works as well as HIIT.

Although you don't need any weights to engage in a HIIT exercise, it can be done using weights, but at the beginning of your journey, we are more interested in your heart rate than how your muscles look or how many steps you can walk.[48,49]

Benefits of High-Intensity Interval Training

- Increase glucose metabolism in the muscles, therefore creating better insulin sensitivity
- Improved blood pressure
- Improved overall cardiovascular health
- Reduction in abdominal fat, therefore lowering triglycerides and cholesterol
- Reduction in body weight

If you are new to exercise, or not a fan, then let me dispel a few concerns you might have before we look at strategies for improving your exercise Pillar.

You don't need to join a gym or have special equipment for HIIT

Simple things like climbing stairs or walking up a steep hill are quick ways of getting your heart rate up. Even everyday chores can be HIIT training like vigorously vacuuming for 10 minutes would do the trick.

You don't need a lot of space to do HIIT

Bodyweight exercises are great for hitting your movement goals and raising your heart rate. You could easily do a bodyweight circuit such as 10 press-ups, 10 air squats, and 10 sit-ups for 5 to 10 minutes. That can all be done in a very small space.

You don't need to exercise for an hour or more to get healthy

How does 30 seconds a day sound? It's true, even if you are new to exercise, adding 30 seconds a day is a great start. You don't need to do hours in the gym, and I personally think, anything over 30 minutes is probably too much. Getting into movement habits is what's important.

If you can do 30 seconds a day, then over time, you can add another 30 and soon you might be doing 5 or 10 minutes. You really don't have to exercise much for HIIT to be effective. You could begin by parking your car farther from your workplace and then walk fast to your office. Maybe take the stairs instead of an elevator. Even these two things would make a difference.

Strategies For Increasing Exercise & Movement

Exercise and movement are a massive subject and I probably won't cover everything here, but here are my top strategies for increasing HIIT.

Exercising for 10 Seconds Multiple Times is Better than Nothing

I know that sounds unbelievable, but it's true. 10 seconds multiple times a day is an effective start. If you are new to movement and exercise and you're not really keen to join a gym or do some type of structured workout, then start small until you can build up to a minimum of 30 seconds a day.

Getting into a movement habit is important and it is going to be supportive to you getting well. So, let's get you going with something like this: anytime you're in a place where you're waiting for something like the microwave to finish, or an elevator to stop, then just start jogging on the spot. You'll be surprised at how fun this can be, and hopefully, after doing 10 seconds for a few days, you'll turn that into 20, then 30 seconds, then a minute. In time, if you build slowly, you'll find you can do 10-15 minutes a day.

Remember, you aren't doing this to win a race, just to get a little out of breath.

Do Short Circuit AMRAPS Rather than Long Slow Exercise

In CrossFit there's an acronym I'd like you to adopt AMRAP – As Many Rounds (or Reps) As Possible. What this means is if you have 10 minutes to spare, then you might do an AMRAP circuit in that time, and it could look like this:

In 10 minutes do As Many Rounds as Possible of:
- 4 Jumping Jacks
- 4 Air Squats (bodyweight squatting without any equipment)
- 4 Press-ups
- 30 Seconds Rest
- Repeat for until time runs out

By doing this type of exercise, you'll work at your own pace, and each time you do this AMRAP you'll have a record of the number of rounds and reps you achieved. You can use that to track your fitness because next time you do this AMRAP you can try and beat your numbers.

If you're new to exercise you can also scale this to your level, so maybe you do 1 or 2 of each exercise in the same time-frame. What makes an AMRAP useful is that if you only have 3, 5 or 15 minutes, you can still do the same exercises but just in different amounts of time. This type of circuit can be done anywhere and is another reason this is a suitable exercise for reversing your condition.

Get a Workout Buddy and Speed Walk at Lunch

If you do want to move more and you only have a short amount of time during your lunch break, then it can be helpful to have a buddy to exercise with. A buddy can make exercising less boring, but it can also add motivation. You'll be able to keep each other accountable and that can help get you going when you'd rather not.

Even though walking isn't that effective for reversing your condition, speed walking is a little different and might look like this: over a period of 10 to 15 minutes you'll alternate your walking pace. First, walk at your normal pace for 30 seconds, then walk as fast as you can for 20 to 30 seconds (or jog if you're able to), rinse and repeat for the time you chose. What you'll find is HIIT walking is a quick and efficient exercise.

Take Up CrossFit

No matter what you've heard about CrossFit, it's an excellent structured activity that will help get you fitter and stronger, while being challenging and fun. A good CrossFit gym will scale every exercise movement to your fitness and ability level. If you can't do a press-up, then the coaches will help scale your exercise until you can. If you're unfit, then the coaches will make sure you can do something at your level to get a good workout while still making progress.

CrossFit is one of the few structured exercises that *is* suitable for all levels, even for people in their 70's and up. The CrossFit's credo on exercise is: 'Constantly varied, functional movement, done with high intensity.' which makes CrossFit ideal for our needs.

A typical CrossFit session starts with a warm-up, then some type of strength activity, then finishes with a 10 to 20-minute HIIT workout, which is in that sweet spot of what we're looking for. You'll also be joining a fantastic community of members who will cheer you on and help you every step of the way. Give it a go, as most gyms will have a free introduction and skills training session.

Get a Jump Rope

Another great exercise if you are short of space and time is jumping rope. This might sound old-school but there isn't much better exercise for getting your heart rate up than a jump rope. I guarantee that 2-5 minutes of jumping rope is going to be all the exercise you need to help make you more insulin sensitive. It's such a good and underrated aerobic exercise and you can do it pretty much anywhere. Also, if you have children, this can be a fun activity for you both.

Create Time in Your Calendar

Too many people have a calendar full of meetings and events which pertain to doing things for others, but they rarely put things in the calendar which leaves room for themselves. If you actively create space for yourself in your calendar, then there's at least a chance you'll use that time for some movement and exercise. You now know you don't need an hour to exercise, so do put something in your calendar, maybe take a few minutes before your lunch to do a 10-

minute AMRAP before you grab some food. Maybe create a calendar reminder and don't just dismiss it when it comes up. Remind yourself this is for your wellbeing and health and skipping this is letting yourself down.

Forget the All-or-Nothing Mentality

I talked about this in Thinking Traps and it's also true for movement and exercise. The best way to approach exercise is with a flexibility which allows you to participate when you can and give yourself a break if you can't. Ideally, you'll have the mindset that you can always find 30 seconds in your day to do some movement when time is tight. Whatever you do, don't go with the all-or-nothing mindset: "*If I can't do 15 minutes then there's no point doing anything.*" It's this type of thought that will get in the way of incremental progress which can sabotage any of the Five Pillars.

If you typically have an all-or-nothing approach, it's time to work on having a little more flexibility, especially when it comes to exercise.

Dump Your Excuses

Honestly, there will be times when you just don't feel up to doing any intense activity. That's fine. This ties into the all-or-nothing thinking and giving yourself a break if you don't have the time or energy to exercise. However, there's a difference between having times when you don't feel up to exercising and the problem of making habitual excuses why you don't exercise.

If you ever engage in that other thinking trap, labeling: "*I'm too old or fat to workout*" or, "*I'm not athletic or strong enough to exercise*", then I'm afraid you're just making excuses. Time and again, I've been clear that even 30 seconds of exercise a day is a good start. You don't have to be strong, athletic, thin, young or gym experienced to do something in the day to raise your heart rate.

Doing yard work counts. Walking the dog up some hills counts. Dancing to your favorite music while you make lunch, counts. Always do something that is suitable to you. Take your time and build up if you don't have stamina. Nobody is judging you but you, so try and be relaxed about it.

Have Realistic Expectations

If you are starting out and adding exercise to your day, then don't aim to do a workout Beyoncé does. Just because an exercise routine is in a magazine, it doesn't mean it's right for you. Doing too much, too soon, can lead to frustration and fatigue. It is always best to ease into movement if you're not fit to let your body get used to moving.

Once you've started slow, your body will adapt, and you'll gain stamina while getting incrementally stronger and fitter. If you start off doing too much, it's easy to get injured or judge yourself harshly if you're not able to keep up or do the activities that some fitness instructor is showing you.

Therefore, I like starting with a few seconds a day as a goal, and each week add a little more. If it takes you a year to build up to 15-minute HIIT exercise, then that is your pace and that's great. Don't judge yourself against what others do or what the media tell you to do. Listen to your body, take your time and above all, enjoy the process.

You Don't Need Money or Equipment to Exercise

I like AMRAP's and I love bodyweight exercises for the simple reason you can do them anywhere and they cost you zero money. There are lots of videos on YouTube on bodyweight exercises (calisthenics) but here are a few of my favorites which you can incorporate into your AMRAP.

Press-ups, bicycle sit-up, crunches, Russian twist, air squats, lunges, planks, glute bridge, burpee, jumping jack, pike and push-ups.

Fun Before Intensity

Even though I want you to do some type of intense activity to raise your heart rate, what we want to do is make sure you enjoy yourself first rather than killing yourself to work more intensely. It's easier to enjoy what you do and build up the intensity as your fitness improves, rather than think you must go all out every time.

If you can enjoy your activity, then you are more likely to continue to do it and build that into a good habit of regular exercise. Think fun, think consistency, and then think intensity to build that habit.

PART THREE:

NUTRITION

"I could talk food all day. I love good food."
— Tom Brady

Nutrition Made Simple

There's so much free information about food, recipes and diets these days that we really are spoiled for choice but not always in a good way. Information on what to eat is often confusing and contradictory. Personally, I don't like the word diet when making nutrition changes to our lifestyle. This is because of all the baggage the word carries with it.

The word diet sounds temporary, something you do for a few weeks, but to cleanse your blood, we're looking at long-term lifestyle and nutrition balancing. Amongst all this information are the headline wars to warn us to avoid fat, cheese, eggs, and red meat while eating more whole grains, pasta, fruit drink and smoothies to get healthy. This information is typically wrong and just thrown at us without any scientific back-up.

Also, if you walk down any aisle, in any store, there's row upon row of food products advertising their health benefits, with claims such as heart healthy, low in sugar, calorie-free, fat-free, organic, gluten-free, protein-added, fortified with vitamins, and on and on. It becomes bewildering to know where to start.

There are also many different diets such as the Paleo diet, Keto diet, South Beach diet, Atkins, Mediterranean, the Zone diet and even the cabbage soup diet. It really is mind-blowing trying to figure out what the best one is to help reverse diabetes, prediabetes or metabolic syndrome. And to a point, all these diets will work for some people, just not everyone. Most of these diets (except maybe Paleo) are usually temporary ways of eating and are not really a sustainable way to eat for the rest of our lives. Sure, you can lose weight eating cabbage soup for a while, but it's not going to reverse your condition, let alone be a satisfying choice for more than a few days.

If you are looking for a way to eat without too much hassle, no gimmicks or expensive proprietary products then you need to cleanse your blood using the Five Pillars approach and learn to choose food that is good for your blood, and still enjoyable.

The approach we'll take is a simple one: moderate protein, moderate fat, and low(ish) carbohydrates mainly from vegetables. By balancing your food this way you'll be providing your body with enough fuel to help it work efficiently without becoming overwhelmed by sugar.

Over the next few pages, we'll look at the best food options for balancing your blood work. Plus, these foods are great for helping you lose weight if that's one of your goals. Then we'll examine the foods choices which you'll need to be a little more cautious with because of how they will impact your insulin and blood sugar. And finally, we'll look at food choices which ideally need to be removed from everyday meals and just saved for the occasional treat, because these food choices will have the highest impact on your blood sugar.

For many of my clients, changing the food they eat and understanding what a healthier option is can be a fun process, because new food choices open a whole new world of meal ideas and fresh new tastes. Many people fall into nutrition ruts, buying the same items week in, week out, and not expanding their meal 'repertoire' or trying anything different. It's not that there's anything wrong with this but often when we get stuck eating the same foods. We often get stuck eating poorly because our brains will naturally encourage us to eat more foods that are carbohydrate-rich. Over time these food choices will contribute to overwhelming your blood with too much sugar.

As much as new food experiences can be fun, there will always be some people who have a tough time eating well and staying consistent with balanced food choices. If this is you, don't worry and don't give up. If you're having a challenging time getting your food choices right daily, just remember - progress not perfection. Small changes here and there will make a difference.

Later in this section, I'll talk about some food alternatives to traditional favorites, which at least might help you stay on track while giving you enough of a difference that you can still enjoy things like pizza but with a blood kind spin to it. All I ask is you keep an open mind and know when changing from old food choices to new food choices it can take time. Use the **Mind Work** section if you find you get stuck with unhelpful thinking about food and the changes you are making.

A quick note about cutting carbs. When I talk about cutting carbs we're not talking about a keto, paleo, or very low carb diet. These approaches can be helpful to a lot of people, and if you want to try these approaches then that's your prerogative, but I generally don't advise people to go from a traditional American diet to a restrictive diet because the change can be too huge. Also, going into a low carbohydrates approach too quickly can seem extremely limiting and ultimately boring. And once boredom sets in it becomes easier to abandon a plan, even if your mindset is good in the beginning.

In your nutrition approach there is always wiggle room in the foods you can choose and there's a place for treat meals (read Exception Eating in **Mind Work**) here and there. This plan isn't supposed to be a rigid experience for you, rather a balanced approach which will make it easy to make small successful changes. I don't subscribe to 'this-is-the-only-one-way' type of eating and I hope you'll find the following nutrition advice simple and easy to follow.

Portion Sizes

Before we look at your food options, I want to go over portions sizes and how to get a good sense of what might be ideal for you. I'm not a fan of weighing but having a simple way to assess if you are eating enough or too much can be valuable in the beginning. The good news is the measuring tool I use is easy to carry around with you – it's your hand.

One of the good things about using your hand as a guide is that it isn't precise, so you don't need to worry about getting fixated on the exact amount. I don't want you to get hung up on precise portions, that's just weird and obsessive. Being a little over or under isn't a problem. If you are close enough, that's good enough. In time you'll instinctively know what a good portion size is.

Full Hand Portion

For main meals, make sure you prioritize protein and make sure you have a good-sized portion. Too often people, especially women, under-eat protein on a regular basis, so I recommend using your full hand as a guide. The good thing about using the hand method is your portion size will scale appropriately with your physical size unless you have the hand size of E.T.

Also, make sure the protein you choose is as *thick* as the side of your hand and larger than your palm but not exceeding the end of your fingertips. This will make a Full Hand portion of steak, chicken, fish and most other proteins, and weighs in at around 4oz to 7oz.

You'll use this Full Hand portion for main meals only.

Palm Portion

A Palm portion is where the protein fits in your palm, from heel of your palm to the start of your fingers. This is generally going to give you around 3-4oz of protein and is the minimum amount of protein you'll want for a main meal or a generous snack.

Cupped Palm Portion

This is when you curl your fingers towards your palm, and you have a little channel running down your palm. This would be around good for something like a snack portion of berries, nuts or jerky.

Double Cupped Hand

This is a great portion for your leafy greens as you have fewer restrictions on these types of food than almost anything else. Essentially, you place both hands together and just curl your fingers up and make a bowl with your hands.

Fist Portion

When you close your hand into a fist, this gives you about a cup size portion which is a sensible size for many of the GO vegetable portions. You never want to have a Fist portion of anything in the WHOA! or NO sections, as that size portion will contain way too many carbs for any of your meals.

Half Fist Portion

As the name suggests, this would be half of the Fist_portion and equates to about half a cup in size. Your Half Fist portion is measured from the bottom two fingers of your fist. This is ideal for WHOA! vegetables and starches.

Two or Three-Finger Portion

This is just like it sounds. If you hold up three fingers, you'll have your three-finger portion. Remove one finger and you have a two finger portion. This is a good guide for WHOA! starches like rice and potato.

This may seem like a small portion for these types of foods, but they contain a lot of carbohydrates. A Three Finger portion is ideal to keep the carbs manageable for your blood.

Two Finger portion is great for a snack-size piece of cheese or jerky.

Finger Tip and Thumb Tip Portion

This portion is from the tip of your finger down to the first knuckle crease and this represents a similar portion size to one teaspoon. And for the thumb, it's the same idea and equates to roughly a tablespoon.

Meal Timing

When I explain meal timings to my clients, I often see the same look on their faces. It's that look that screams: "Are you crazy?" I guess around 90% of my clients don't eat enough food. Most come to me after trying many other diets to get healthy, and a lot of these diets are based on calorie counting or fasting or drinking shakes.

By now you know calorie counting is a bad idea and so is calorie deficit eating. The more balanced food you can eat, the fuller and more satiated you'll feel, while having more energy. Who wouldn't want to eat more if those are the benefits?

Eat Every Three Hours

I don't impose many rules on my clients (or you) but this is one I'd like you to try and follow more closely than not. Eating every three hours is important, and these regular intervals will not only control your blood sugar throughout the day, but we need to make sure you're eating enough so you don't find yourself hungry. Getting hungry is a sure way of sabotaging good intentions. We make bad food choices when hungry, so avoiding that is important.

A lot of my clients are used to eating only three meals a day, and some even skip meals because they claim to not have time to eat in their busy work schedule. But if we don't eat enough then we're letting one of our Five Pillars come crashing down and that goes against everything we need to do for balance.

Typically, a person's stomach will empty between two to four hours after eating if they're eating a balanced meal of primarily protein and fat with a little carb. However, if somebody eats a meal containing more fruit and carbohydrate foods then these items go through the digestive system in as little as fifty minutes, which is why, if you have a carb snack like chips or a muffin, within an hour you're hungry again.

Foods containing fat and protein will always take longer to digest, therefore you'll feel fuller for longer and if you're eating every three hours, there's less chance of tipping into hunger and making unhealthy food choices.

Also, don't take 'eating every three hours' as eating a big meal every three hours. Instead we'll be adding snacks throughout the day until you're eating around 6 meals a day. Ideally, I want you to aim for this type of scenario: breakfast, snack, lunch, snack, dinner, snack.

You might find your schedule means you have to play with this order a little, but essentially six meals a day is the goal (or maybe seven if you have a long day). I've worked with people who work shifts and their meal timings look more like this: dinner, snack, snack, lunch, snack, breakfast. Whichever way you choose to eat, having more regular food is going to support you throughout the day and will have a positive effect on your blood, mood, cognition and energy levels.

Eat Protein and/or Fat at Every Meal

Now you know about portions, our next step to minimize insulin release in your body is to make sure you prioritize protein and fat over carbohydrates anytime you eat. Because you'll be eating around six times a day, each meal will need to include some type of protein and/or fat. I say and/or because something food such as cheese contains primarily fat, but it also contains a little protein. You could eat two mozzarella sticks for a snack and that would be a fat and a protein mix. But if you had a Full Palm of chicken, then that would be protein only. Either way, a protein and/or a fat meal is going to fuel you without the spikes in blood sugar and insulin.

Protein and fat also take longer to digest, which will get you through that three-hour window between meals and give you increased energy through that time. This a win-win for your blood and body when it comes to food.[52]

Why Skipping Meals is a Bad Idea

Something serial dieters and people desperate to lose weight often do is skip meals. The idea behind it can usually be traced back to the calorie counting nonsense, with the less you eat, the more weight you'll lose. But skipping meals is a terrible idea. For you to cleanse your blood you need nutritional help, not sabotage. When skipping meals, you're setting yourself up for failure.

I know for me, when I'm hungry I'm more likely to grab an unhealthy snack or order an off-plan meal. Apart from this, there are more significant reasons for not skipping meals. Skipping meals has been linked to an increase in metabolic syndrome, including an increased waist circumference, insulin resistance, cardiovascular risk and nonalcoholic fatty liver disease.[67,68]

This alone should be enough to encourage you to make sure you eat regularly throughout the day; but just to reinforce how important eating regularly is, studies have shown that eating more frequently increases insulin sensitivity (one of our primary goals), lowers LDL cholesterol and waist circumference.[69,70,71]

For far too long, dietary guidelines have only focused on what food to eat but the importance of how frequently to eat hasn't been a priority. From my experiences with clients, they are far happier and more successful in reversing their condition (and losing weight) by eating more frequently than they ever did skipping meals or counting calories.

In the beginning of eating every three hours it's quite usual to feel full and not want to eat. This is usually a temporary experience, and as long as you keep at it (don't stuff food down if you really can't) your body soon adapts to your new way of eating. Something wonderful happens at this point. Your blood becomes cleaner and when the body knows it has a good regular source of fuel from protein and fat, it can then stop spending so much time cleaning your blood and can start to burn body fat for fuel rather than all the excess glucose floating around.

In time, by eating every three hours, your body recognizes this frequent fueling window and adapts accordingly. You'll also find your hunger hormones will start working correctly again. You'll recognize when you are hungry and full as ghrelin and leptin do their job. This in turn, will help to ultimately lower your carb intake and keep your blood glucose and insulin levels down.

Don't Skip Breakfast

If skipping meals is going to hinder your progress, then skipping breakfast is going to make things even harder. I don't know about you, but I love breakfast so much so that I look forward to breakfasting the moment I wake. It's probably my favorite meal of the day. However, I know there are many people who don't like breakfast or skip it because they're busy getting ready for work or just don't like eating first thing in the morning.

I understand both reasons, but I would encourage you to work on prioritizing this meal because it does set your body up for the day. If we have a good amount of protein and fat for breakfast the benefits we gain from this will be better appetite control through the day, a reduction in ghrelin (hunger hormone), reduced poor food decision-making (including grabbing quick and usually sugary snacks through the day), and less unhealthy snacking at night. All that from a good breakfast.[72,73,74]

By a good protein and fat breakfast, I'm talking mainly about things like bacon and eggs; or a cheddar, bacon and spinach omelet. When you go through the **What to Eat** list shortly, start thinking about how you are going to make sure you give yourself more time in the morning to get a good breakfast into your body.

Food Choices

To begin balancing your nutrition, we're going to start with what I call GO food choices. These are your everyday go-to food items. Anything in this list can be had multiple times a day and in any combination. You can eat any of these foods until you feel physically satisfied, which doesn't mean you eat until you pass out because we can still eat too much of a good thing.

Also, if your ghrelin and leptin hormones have been out of balance for a long time you might find you're not quite aware of when you are full until you get to that 'stuffed' feeling. However, once you start reducing carbs and sugar, you'll start to retrain your body and soon your ghrelin and leptin hormones will switch back on and you'll be more aware of when you're full and need to refuel.

If you stick close to the sensible portions I outline below, then you'll be fine.

GO Proteins

Meat & Poultry

Beef (all cuts)	Pork
Bison & Buffalo	Turkey (inc. Turkey Bacon)
Chicken	Venison & other game
Duck & other game birds	
Lamb	
Liver (all types)	

Seafood

Clams	Scallops
Crab	Shrimp
Fish (all types)	Snails
Lobster	Squid
Mussels	

Other GO Proteins

Bone Broth
Deli Meat*
Egg Whites
Protein Powders
Tofu

*A little more processed than I'd like, but generally okay.

GO Protein Portions (Recommended)

These are your main sources of protein and you have a lot more leeway here than with almost anything else. Even if you eat a little more protein than you need, it won't make much of a difference to your blood or weight.

A main meal portion size of protein is typically going to be a Full Hand portion. This means, if the protein you choose fills all or most of the whole of your hand, then that's a big enough portion for you. For a snack size portion of protein, you'll be looking at anywhere between a Two Finger portion all the way up to a Palm portion. If you're wondering about egg whites, which are an excellent protein, around a

Fist portion (or a cup size if you need to use a container) would be about the same amount of protein as a Full Hand of chicken.

One of the best and easiest proteins on this list is bone broth, which has a fantastic amount of protein. You can use this as a snack or as an addition to a main meal if you need to increase your protein a little. A cup of bone broth is about the same amount of protein as half a chicken breast. Bone broth is different from standard broth. Bone broth has a lot of protein, whereas standard broth tends to be more like flavored water and contains minimal protein. Standard broth is something you can drink as an alternative to tea or for added water (in the Go Liquid section below), but it isn't a protein substitute.

GO Carbohydrates

Vegetables

Artichokes	Leafy Greens (all types)
Asparagus	Lettuce (all types)
Broccoli	Mushrooms
Brussels Sprouts	Okra
Cabbage	Onions (all varieties)
Cauliflower	Peppers (all varieties)
Celery	Snap Peas
Cucumbers	Tomatoes
Green Beans	Yellow Squash
Jicama	Zucchini (inc. Zucchini Noodles)

Fruits

Lemon
Lime

GO Carbohydrates Portions (Recommended)

A main meal portion from this list is typically a Fist Size portion unless it's a leafy green like lettuce, and then you can eat a Double Cupped Hand portion or more without any concerns.

All these vegetables can be combined, and they all add good fiber. It doesn't matter how you cook them, so find your favorite way and have fun.

Lemons and limes are great to use in water to add flavor or over salad, so use them as you see fit.

GO Fats

Hard & Soft Fats

> Avocado (inc. Avocado Oil)
> Butter (inc. Ghee)
> Coconut Cream
> Coconut Oil
> Eggs
> Hard Cheeses (Cheddar, Colby, Gouda etc.)
> Heavy & Heavy Whipping Cream
> Olives (inc. Olive Oils)
> Semi-Soft Cheeses (Mozzarella, Goats Cheese etc.)
> Soft Cheese (Cottage, Ricotta)
> Sour Cream

GO Fat Portions (Recommended)

Fats are a little trickier to measure as they can be different substances, solid or liquid. However, if you're eating fats from the GO section, then you really can't go wrong. A typical portion of cheese can be the size of One or Two Fingers. Many kinds of cheese come in premade sticks, and I find them useful to have in the fridge for when I need a quick snack, or I find I'm hungrier than normal. A stick can often keep me going until my next meal. I find mozzarella sticks to be one of my favorites.

Half an avocado is a good portion of fat to have as either a snack or in conjunction with a main meal. I'll often mix an avocado with some coriander and lime to make guacamole and add that to my protein.

Other good fat portions are 2-4 eggs for any meal, and 2 eggs as a snack. I have mine with salt and if I'm feeling feisty, a little sriracha;

and before you ask, there isn't a limit on the number of eggs you can eat in a day. Although, I don't recommend going the Paul Newman route from the movie 'Cool Hand Luke' and eat fifty at one time.

Coconut oil is tasty and versatile with a good Thumb Tip portion, something you could add to coffee, just eat raw or cook with. The same goes for sour cream, a Thumb Tip portion is a good dollop.

GO Liquids

Hot & Cold

> Broth
> Tea (Herbal, Green, Unsweetened Ice Tea)
> Water (Sparkling, Plain, Naturally Flavored)

GO Liquid Portions (Recommended)

All these options are fine to add to your 80-100oz a day. Tea without caffeine is good and remember to check out the tips for drinking more water in the Five Pillars section if you struggle with drinking enough.

WHOA! Food Choices

WHOA! Food choices are where we need to be a little more cautious. If you've ever ridden a horse, in the beginning, one of the things you learn is to say WHOA! to slow down your horse, otherwise, it's easy to lose control – and it's the same with food. With WHOA! foods you're probably looking at smaller portions than you'd typically have, and you'll eat them less often.

WHOA! foods are what I call 'fillers' – portions of food to fill you up and make the meal look bigger and more substantial by adding things like rice or potatoes. These are the types of foods which are generally cheaper than protein, and over the years have taken over our plates.

The other thing to remember with WHOA! foods is they do contain a higher amount of carbohydrates than our GO foods and it's easy to get carried away with portions. Because these are fillers, it's easy to end up eating 2-3 portions of a WHOA! food in a single meal without realizing.

It's not that WHOA! foods are bad choices, it's just that if we're not cautious with our portions we can eat an amazing amount of carbs very quickly, and this turns not-so-bad-food into an overwhelming barrage of sugar in your blood.

WHOA! Protein

Yogurt, Meat & Poultry

> Greek Yogurt (5%, 2%, 0%)
> Bacon (Pork varieties)
> Sausages (inc. Chicken)
> Jerky (unflavored - watch for hidden sugar)

WHOA! Protein Portions (Recommended)

WHOA! proteins are not bad choices, but we do need to be a little more cautious about these choices than GO proteins. I love bacon and could eat a lot of it but do try and keep bacon to around three strips as a portion. A little more now and then isn't a problem, but the high saturated fat and salt in bacon can make this a less than ideal choice. Not because it will affect your heart or your blood, but because it can affect your bowels, and getting blocked up back there is no fun. However, bacon is still a tasty choice and one you can have daily if you wish, so turn that frown upside down and enjoy bacon in moderation.

Another protein to be cautious with are sausages, only because most store-bought sausages contain a surprising amount of carbs. I know there are many different types of sausage and there will be some of better quality and lower carb varieties than others but just to be safe all types: chicken-apple, pork, beef or any other variation - needs a little prudence.

A typical sausage size is about 5-6 inches, so you want to keep a portion to about two sausages max unless you know the quality is good and doesn't contain carb fillers. If your sausages are a little smaller, like breakfast sausage, then around four would be fine. I'm a fan of the Jimmy Dean range of natural sausages as they contain very little carbs.

Greek yogurt is a hybrid food as it is primarily protein but does contain carbs, so if you have it as a snack, then a single pot (4-6oz) is big enough. If you want to add some yogurt on top of one of your meals or on the side, then a Two Finger portion would be adequate as an additional protein.

WHOA! Carbohydrates

Many people are under the illusion that they can eat a lot of fruit in a day, but you now know better, right? If you remember, there was a big campaign to encourage people to eat 5 pieces of fruit or veg a day. The problem with that guideline is that most people prefer eating fruit because it's sweeter, so 5-a-day fruit or veg typically became 4 fruits and one veg, which is terrible for your blood. WHOA! carbs can get high quickly, so keep the portions sizes small, and don't combine veg from this section.

Also, *one* fruit a day is the best limit to go for, unless you have berries and then you can have a Cupped Palm twice a day.

Vegetables & Beans

Barley	Potatoes (all varieties)
Beets	Quinoa
Carrots	Rice (all varieties)
Corn	Squashes (Winter, Buternut etc.)
Garden Peas	
Legumes/Beans (all varieties)	
Lentils (all varieties)	

Fruits

Apples	Melon (all varieties)
Banana (small or half)	Oranges
Berries (all varieties)	Papaya
Cuties, Manderins, Clementines	Pears
Figs (fresh only)	Pineapple
Grapefruit	Stone Fruits (Apricots, Plums,
Grapes	Mango, Peaches, etc.)
Kiwi	

WHOA! Carbohydrates Portions (Recommended)

All carbohydrates in this section have the potential to turn into NO foods just because of portion sizes. Typically, the portions of food in this section are usually way too big, especially in restaurants, so we need to learn to use these foods sensibly and curb our portion sizes to make these foods okay for our blood.

If you remember, fruit is still just sugar (fructose) and fiber, so again I'm going to remind you, limit your fruit to one piece a day. That portion is for all fruit except berries. What I like to do is take 2 Cupped Palm portions of berries and split them throughout the day, that way I can enjoy a little fruit more often. In fact, splitting portions is something you can do this with most fruit. This is a great way of reducing carbs in one sitting, while still getting the taste and enjoyment from fruit. Whichever way you choose to eat fruit, get used to seeing fruit as 'Natures Candy', rather than as a healthy food option.

With vegetables and starches, go with a Half Fist portion just because these foods are still quite high in carbs, so limiting the portion makes them more reasonable for your plan. One thing you might be surprised to see when you serve up your WHOA! carbs in sensible portions is how small the portion might be compared to what you're probably used to, especially with such options as corn and carrots. In the beginning, you might find your smaller portions not as satisfying, but once you get used to eating this way and you're filling up on protein and fats, these smaller portions will be enough.

WHOA! Fats

Soft Cheeses & Nuts

> Soft Cheeses (Brie, Camembert, Cream Cheese etc)
> Nuts (all varieties)
> Nut Butters (Peanut, Almond etc. - watch for extra sugar varieties)

WHOA! Fat Portions (Recommended)

Fats make food taste great, and these three WHOA! fats are some of my personal favorite foods. Fat based food make ideal as snacks because they're a mix of protein, fat, and carbs. Most people are surprised to know that nuts tend to be equal parts protein and carbohydrates but with a higher amount of fat as the main macronutrient.

Although I love nuts, they still need to be eaten sparingly. A good portion of nuts would be a Cupped Hand portion for a snack, and you could have this twice a day if you wish. Nut butter would be around a 1-2 Thumb Tip portion, although, for full transparency, I do have a larger spoonful before bed.

Soft cheeses are still good to have for snacks or an accompaniment to a main meal. A good Thumb Tip or two is fine and I especially like cream cheese spread down the center of celery as a snack.

WHOA! Liquids

Soft & Hard Drinks

Alternative Unsweetened Milks (Almond, Coconut, Soy etc.)
Beer (all brands)
Coffee (Black or w/ Cream or Half & Half)
Diet or Zero Sodas (all varieties)$
Milk (all cow or goat varieties)
Liquor/Spirits (Whiskey, Vodka, Gin etc.)
Sports Drinks (no sugar varieties - Powerade, Red Bull)$
Tea (black with or without milk)
Wine (red, white, sparkling or rose)

$Research shows artificial sweeteners can increase appetite, so use with caution and sparingly.[75,76]

WHOA! Liquid Portions (Recommended)

I recommend not having more than one of these drinks in a day, except maybe coffee and tea, although try to keep these to around 2-3 cups a day max. This is mainly because caffeine can impact on your sleep. Even if you think it doesn't affect your sleep, it will. I caution you to minimize milk as much as you can as it does contain a high amount of carbs, which makes it another borderline WHOA!/NO food choice. Unfortunately, all these liquids don't count towards your daily intake of 100oz as I want you to get used to making water your main way to hydrate enough through the day.

    Alcohol is also a tough one. Personally, I would like to put all alcohol in the NO section because it has many negative effects on the body and it's easily overused. However, if you are sensible with wine and spirits, and stick to only one drink per day then you can keep it in this section. If you're likely to want more than one drink per day, then this goes into the NO section. Alcohol is far too easy to overdo, and when your inhibitions are lowered, the decision-making process is affected. Making choices after drinking alcohol means you're at risk of eating off-plan foods from the NO section. You know what I mean if you've ever had a few drinks and decided pizza covered in mac and cheese would be the best thing in the world to eat at midnight.

Start seeing alcohol for what it is: beer is essentially liquid bread and wine liquid grapes, making these two choices more in line with NO food choices. Spirits on the other hand, are a little different because most of the sugar is removed in distillation, therefore spirits are naturally low in carbs and won't have the same impact on your blood sugar as beer and wine. However, I caution you, spirits are higher in alcohol content which can still lead to unhealthy food choices. Even if you switch to spirits, stick to one serving a day.

Diet soda is full of artificial sugar and that's something we still need to minimize. One diet soda a day in the beginning is generally okay, but if you're a big soda drinker learn to transition over to something like sparkling water if it's the fizzy experience you enjoy.

WHOA! Miscellaneous

Alternative Flours (Almond, Coconut etc.)
Condiments (all types)
Dark Chocolate (70%+ cocoa value)
Jam/Jelly (sugar-free varieties)
Oatmeal (steelcut & unflavored)
Splenda, Stevia & Other Sweeteners[$]

[$]Research shows artificial sweeteners can increase appetite, so use sparingly.[75,76]

WHOA! Miscellaneous Portions (Recommended)

I think it goes without saying all these items should be used in moderation. Condiments are full of hidden sugar, so keep to no more than a Finger Tip portion and you'll be okay. Oatmeal is very high in carbs, but it is also a good fiber, so I'll leave it in this section for now. Just make sure you have about a Half Fist portion (dry) and have it with water. You can always top it off with a little heavy cream to make it creamier. Just don't make it with all milk as that adds a lot of carbs on top of the oats which can push this into a NO option.

A square or two of a superior quality chocolate now and then is also acceptable when you feel you want something chocolaty or dessert-like. Just make sure you stick to that portion.

If you like to bake, then you might find challenges in this area, as all traditional baked goods are a NO. If you can use the alternative flours then that's a good step forward, but ideally, if it's a baked food don't put it on your plate.

NO Food Choices

Finally, we come to the food choices which will contribute to your current condition. These are foods high in carbohydrates and sugars and just plain bad if eaten daily. As I've said before, you can have anything you choose, as you have free will, but eating food from the NO list will have negative consequences on your blood. Foods from the NO section are going to lead to higher glucose and insulin in your blood and if you want to reverse your condition, removing these items is going to make a significant difference to your overall health.

One of the first nutrition priorities you'll have if you're going to cleanse your blood is learning to leave these NO foods alone. As hard as that might seem in the beginning, it pays off in the long-run.

The food choices listed below are often our favorite foods (mainly because they give the brain a happy high), so I'm okay with you saving some of these items for special occasions or as a sometime treat, but they should not be viewed as daily choices anymore. The sooner you get past that internal disappointment and tantrum (I know you'll have one as soon as you read the list) and be adult about your food choices, the healthier you're going to be.

NO Protein

None. Nada. Zip. Zilch. Basically, there are no NO proteins.

NO Carbohydrates

General Starches

Flour (wheat or corn varieties)
French Fries
Grits
Pasta (all types)
Polenta
Noodles (egg, wheat etc.)

Baked Goods

Baked Goods (Brownies, Cakes, Croissants, Muffins etc.)
Cookies & Biscuits
Bread (all types inc. Pitta)
Crackers (all types)
Tortilla (corn or wheat)
Waffles or Pancakes

Fruits

Canned Fruit (in juice or syrup)
Dried Fruit (Raisins, Figs, Banana etc.)

NO Carbohydrates Cautions

Where to start with these choices? If you think about your typical day of eating, ask yourself how much, and how often, do you eat food from this section? My guess is you have at least two or more portions from this list. It's not unusual to eat bread or baked goods in the morning. In many ways, these foods have just become part of the fabric of our lives, choices that are just there. You might also find yourself eating French fries at lunch, maybe a cookie in the afternoon and pasta for dinner. I won't go into macros for this but just know, if you ate close to what I just mentioned in a day, you're dumping around 45 sugar cubes into your blood.

Yep, I said 45 sugar cubes into your blood. I challenge you to go and eat 45 sugar cubes and not feel sick. This is the sad reality of eating foods from this section that is rarely explained.

I like treats and talk about this in 'Exception Eating' in the **Mind Work** section but a treat doesn't mean it's an anything-goes-blow-out. A treat of bread might be one burger in its bun now and then, or a taco, or a pancake for Sunday brunch. A treat is not 3 or 4 of these things at the same time. Also, I'm fine if you have 3 or 4 fries for taste now and then if you're out at a restaurant and it's not a treat day, because that small amount won't cause too much of a problem. Often having a taste of something you like should be enough to satisfy the urge to have a whole portion. However, be careful those little portions for taste don't trigger you. If it does, go and re-read the 'Trigger Foods' section in the **Mind Work**.

NO Liquids

Soft & Hard Drinks

> Cocktails (inc. fruit juice)
> Fruppaccino (or any syrup milky ice drink)
> Fruity Alcoholic Drinks
> Fruit or Vegetable Smoothies
> Fruit Juice (all types)
> Milky Coffee (Latte, Cappuccino, Mocha etc)
> Sports Drinks (full sugar varieties - Gatorade, Red Bull, Powerade)

NO Liquid Cautions

These are some of the worst things you can put into your body. Most people don't realize how much sugar these drinks contain. For example, if you have a something like a Grande Latte from Starbucks in the morning, followed by 2 cokes during the day, a fruit juice at lunch and an iced tea at dinner, you've just ingested around 38 sugar cubes!!!! I'm not kidding.

So, if you combine that with the amount of NO carbs I mention in the paragraphs above, you might be ingesting the equivalent of 78 sugar cubes in a day and that is absolutely murdering your blood. Seriously, most of these liquids should have a health warning attached to them.

Companies like Starbucks, Dunkin' Donuts, and other coffee establishments are the new fast-food joints. I would bet most people who buy milky coffee have no idea how much sugar is in a drink. Also listing the calorie amount on the menu is ridiculous. What they need to show is the actual sugar content, and then people might start paying attention to how bad these types of drinks are.

Your withdrawal from all these liquids really needs to be the highest priority if you want to cleanse your blood quickly. Eating well while still sticking sugar liquids in your body will make the entire process not only slower, but it might even make your chance of reversing your blood condition next to impossible.

Cocktails and fruity alcoholic drinks (alcopops) are to be avoided completely. Not entirely due to the alcohol content (because most of them are made with spirits and we know that's in the WHOA! section), but because cocktails and fruity alcopops are mixed with fruit juices and sugar. It's far too easy to drink a big cocktail – and by doing so, you'll be ingesting a boatload of sugar in one go. In many cases, there's as much sugar in a fruity alcopops drink as a full sugar soda. Both are off the table if you're to get healthy.

If you don't change anything else about how you eat, change how you drink, and you'll be saving your body from a whole lot of problems.

NO Fats

Mostly from Unhealthy Oils

Margarine (all varieties)
Vegetable Oils

NO Fat Cautions

It can be hard to remove all trans fats from our nutritional choices, as often we aren't sure of the type of oil used to cook or bake certain foods unless it says on the label. If there was a category below NO, then trans fats would be in that category. There's nothing good in trans fats and they directly contribute to obesity, diabetes, cancer and pretty much every disease that can kill you.[77]

Trans fats can be found naturally in animal products like beef, pork, lamb, and butter but I wouldn't worry about this because it does come from a natural source. However, it's how trans fats or trans fatty acids are used in products like margarine, baked goods, cereals, cookies, chips, candy and even in salad dressing and other processed foods that we need to avoid.

Trans fats are a vegetable oil turned into a solid by adding hydrogen atoms which were primarily developed because of the misguided fear of saturated fats, starting back in the 1950's. Luckily, since 2006, the FDA has made it a federal law that manufacturers have to show on a label how much trans fat is included in a product. And because research has shown how bad trans fats are for us, less is being used - but less doesn't mean none.

Long story short, avoid trans fat as much as you can.

NO Miscellaneous

Breakfast Bars (all types)
BBQ Sauces
Candy (all types)
Cereal (all types inc. Granola)
Chips (all types inc. Vegetable Chips in a bag)
Chocolate under 70%
Jelly & Jam (full-sugar types)
Popcorn (yes, popcorn!)
Pretzels
Rice Crackers & Rice Cakes

NO Miscellaneous Cautions

These items are full of sugar and trans fat. And I'm sure you don't need me to tell you how unhealthy they are (but I will anyway). You'll notice BBQ sauce is added here, that's because it contains so much sugar. It's pretty much all sugar. Plus, the amount that usually goes over food is ridiculous. As with other condiments, a Finger Tip portion is a good compromise but if you're used to getting BBQ ribs covered in BBQ sauce, just go with a dry rub and maybe a tiny amount of sauce on the side for taste.

Two Week Meal Plan

All meal plans are subjective. You might like different food than me, so I don't want you to think you can only eat what I've put in this plan. What I would suggest is that you approach this plan as a flexible roadmap to getting into good habits. Take the foods you know to be good and combine them in ways that suites you best.

Typically, the first two weeks are always the hardest, but soon you'll have a better idea of what it takes to stick to your plan and eat well. Does this mean you'll have everything nailed down after two weeks? Absolutely not. But once you can get past the initial sugar withdrawal your food choices will become so much easier.

This plan is going to be basic at first because I like my new clients to start easy and choose options that require less fuss and preparation. Then, once you think you've got the hang of eating well, you can get as creative as you like.

I don't know what your experience of diets has been, but I want you to know eating well and cleansing your blood is not boring. There are several good cookbooks out there based on low-carb eating which have some fantastic recipes. Two of my favorite low-carb food authors are George Stella and Maria Emmerich who have written some enjoyable books which I use regularly.

Most of the meals below are simple to make and don't need much instruction, however, I do have a few food alternatives in the meal plans which I've highlighted with a *.

Alternative recipes can be found in the Finding Substitutes for Your Favorite Foods section.

Monday – Week One

Breakfast:

2-3 x whole eggs with a Cupped Palm of cheese, a Fist of spinach and 3-5 slices of turkey bacon.

Snack:

A medium apple and 8-12 almonds.

Lunch:

Chicken Caesar with added avocado (no croutons). Dressing is fine.

Snack:

Cupped Palm dry roasted edamame.

Dinner:

Steak with half a baked sweet potato. Double Cupped Hand of mixed leafy greens. 1 Thumb Tip of reduced-sugar tomato ketchup.

Snack:

2 Thumb Tips of almond or peanut butter.

Tuesday - Week One

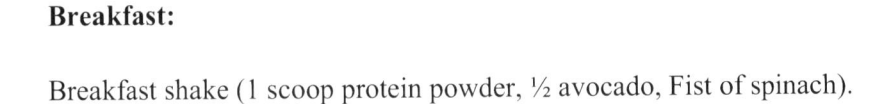

Breakfast:

Breakfast shake (1 scoop protein powder, ½ avocado, Fist of spinach).

Snack:

½ pack roasted seaweed strips with ½ avocado.

Lunch:

A large Palm of tuna mayo and avocado salad.

Snack:

2 or 3 x celery and hummus (spread cream cheese down the center of the celery).

Dinner:

Spicy sausage in a pasta sauce over zucchini noodles.

Snack:

Sugar-free jello with 3 Fingers of Greek yogurt.

Wednesday - Week One

Breakfast:

Jimmy Dean sausage breakfast bowl.

Snack:

Cupped Palm of mixed nuts.

Lunch:

Chicken curry over roast cauliflower.

Snack:

Goat cheese stuffed pepper (half a roasted pepper and spoon in plain or herb goat cheese into the middle).

Dinner:

Pork steaks with Dijon mustard and roast cauliflower.

Snack:

Protein drink with a dash of heavy cream.

Thursday - Week One

Breakfast:

3-4 Jimmy Dean pork sausage links and mushroom omelet.

Snack:

2 x mozzarella sticks and half a banana or small apple.

Lunch:

Bowl of chili with Cupped Palm of cheese & Thumb Tip of sour cream.

Snack:

Cupped Palm of jerky.

Dinner:

Meatballs with Half Fist of rice and roasted asparagus.

Snack:

1-2 x Jimmy Dean fully cooked turkey sausage patties.

Friday - Week One

Breakfast:

4-6oz of Greek yogurt with Cupped Palm of blueberries.

Snack:

Cupped Palm of macadamia nuts.

Lunch:

Cobb salad.

Snack:

2 or 3 x cream cheese celery and salami slices (spread a Thumb Tip of cheese down the center of the celery).

Dinner:

Grilled shrimp and chicken with sweet potato mash.

Snack:

2 Fingers of Colby cheese.

Saturday - Week One

Breakfast:

Almond milk oatmeal with chia, hemp seeds and almond butter (add a Thumb Tip of chia seeds and hemp seeds into the oatmeal and let a Thumb Tip of nut butter melt in the middle).

Snack:

Cupped Palm of mixed nuts.

Lunch:

Philly cheesesteak protein style which means no bread and served on a bed of lettuce.

Snack:

2-3 hardboiled eggs.

Dinner:

Pepperoni and spinach meatzza*. (* in the Substitute section following this Meal Plan)

Snack:

3 x slices of turkey deli meat or turkey bacon.

Sunday - Week One

Breakfast:

Bulletproof coffee (blend cup of fresh coffee with Thumb Tip of coconut oil or MCT oil & Thumb Tip of ghee until frothy).

Snack:

Cupped Palm of mixed nuts.

Lunch:

Roast chicken with mixed roast vegetables and gravy.

Snack:

Cupped Palm dry roasted edamame (try the wasabi!).

Dinner:

Steak on a bed of baby spinach with baked sweet potato fries (from a small potato) with garlic aioli sauce.

Snack:

Protein drink with a dash of heavy cream.

Monday – Week Two

Breakfast:

Classic bacon and eggs your way, with 3 Jimmy Dean pork links.

Snack:

4-5 Cheesy cheddar chips (mix Fist of grated cheese and Finger Tip of sriracha. Place into small chips sizes and bake for 10 mins at 350f on parchment paper until golden).

Lunch:

Beef burrito bow with 3 Fingers of rice, lettuce, cheese, pico de gallo, 2 Fingers of guacamole.

Snack:

4-6oz pot of Greek yogurts with Cupped Palm of blueberries.

Dinner:

Zucchini spaghetti (mince beef in pasta sauce over zucchini noodles).

Snack:

2 Thumb Tips of almond or peanut butter.

Tuesday - Week Two

Breakfast:

Fist of Homemade Granola*

Snack:

Cupped Palm of macadamia nuts.

Lunch:

1-2 cheeseburgers (no bun) with vegetables and salsa.

Snack:

2 x deviled eggs.

Dinner:

Chicken Alfredo over zucchini noodles.

Snack:

Protein drink

Wednesday - Week Two

Breakfast:

Homemade oatmeal* and 2 x bacon.

Snack:

2 x Turkey and cream cheese roll-ups (1-3 slices of turkey with a Thumb Tip of cream cheese spread, then roll it up).

Lunch:

Garlic aioli chicken wrap (4-6 slices of chicken deli meat in a lettuce wrap with aioli).

Snack:

Cupped Palm cantaloupe with Half Fist Greek yogurt.

Dinner:

Sesame beef stir fry with Half Fist of Jasmin rice.

Snack:

Small pot Greek yogurt mixed with Finger Tip of sugar-free jelly.

Thursday - Week Two

Breakfast:

Breakfast shake (1 scoop protein, ½ avocado, Fist of spinach).

Snack:

Cupped Palm of macadamia nuts with 3 strawberries.

Lunch:

4-6 grilled or baked chicken wings and a side salad, 2 mozzarella sticks, Medium apple.

Snack:

2 Fingers of cheddar cheese.

Dinner:

Chicken stir-fry with a variety of chopped veg.

Snack:

1-2 Thumb Tips of almond or peanut butter.

Friday - Week Two

Breakfast:

4-6oz pot of cottage cheese with a Cupped Palm of berries or melon.

Snack:

3-4 sliced peppers and cucumber with hummus dip.

Lunch:

1-2 Bacon cheeseburgers (no bun) with avocado salad.

Snack:

2 x celery with 1-2 Fingers of cheese and 2 sq. of 70% dark chocolate.

Dinner:

Grilled salmon with roast green beans and peppers.

Snack:

4-6oz pot of Greek yogurt mixed with Finger Tip of sugar-free jelly.

Saturday - Week Two

Breakfast:

Protein smoothie (1 scoop protein powder, big dollop of Greek yogurt, Thumb Tip of flax seed meal, Thumb Tip peanut butter, dash heavy cream).

Snack:

2 x mozzarella sticks.

Lunch:

Lamb shawarma salad.

Snack:

Cupped Palm of jerky.

Dinner:

Pesto chicken cheezza*.

Snack:

1-2 Thumb Tips of almond or peanut butter.

Sunday - Week Two

Breakfast:

Italian sausage frittata with 1 x slice of Ezekiel toast and butter.

Snack:

½ pack roasted seaweed strips with ½ avocado.

Lunch:

Bacon and goats cheese salad.

Snack:

Cupped Palm of jerky.

Dinner:

Texas dry rub ribs with coleslaw and 5-8 fries.

Snack:

1-2 Thumb Tips of almond or peanut butter.

There you go, two weeks of delicious meals and a guide I hope you can follow. Remember, you don't have to have exactly what I've put here. You can substitute or switch things around to whatever suits you but do not deviate too far from the types of food and combinations I've listed.

You can download this meal plan at drewcoster.com/worksheets

Substitutes for Your Favorite Foods

You may look at the meal plans or food lists and discovered many foods you love have been relegated to the NO section of the plan. I understand this may cause concerns but I'm here to give you some viable alternatives to enjoy.

For me, I love pizza. However, the carb content in the pizza base is something I need to avoid, so does that mean I can't have pizza ever again? Not a chance. Because pizza is life, I needed to find an alternative and that's where the cheezza and meatzza come into play.

I enjoy the new alternatives to pizza way more than the regular version, so I encourage you to give them a go. These alternatives may not be 100% the best choices you could make to cleanse your blood, but they are items which I'm okay with you adding to your nutrition. It's better to have a little wiggle room in your food choices, rather than being too rigid and feeling deprived.

Because these are alternatives, you might find it takes a little experimentation to get a taste you enjoy. Also, remember these are healthy alternatives to NO favorites and it's unlikely the alternative will taste the same as the original. But who knows, you might find you prefer them in time.

Also, don't give up if the first try doesn't go to plan. Some recipes took me three or four attempts until I found the right variation I liked.

Pizza

Talking about pizza. The easiest compromise is to eat all the topping and maybe a little bit of the crust for taste. The topping is usually a good option for most carnivores as it's mainly meat and cheese, and both are on plan. The base really is a NO, but a small bite or two of crust is going to be okay if you really want it. The crust tends to have a little more flavor than the rest of the doughy base, so one mouthful might be a good alternative.

Other than that, I really like meatzza or cheezza pizza base options. This is where the base is made of either ground beef or turkey for the meatzza and cheese base for cheezza. The recipes are easy, and I think you might love the outcome.

I make the cheezza more than the meatzza just because it's a little easier, but both are just as good. Once you've made these alternative bases, you just make your pizza how you normally would with a tomato base and cover with your favorite toppings.

Meatzza Base

- Take 1lb of ground beef and mix together with 2 eggs.
- Season to taste and spread pizza-thinly onto a baking pan or skillet.
- Bake at 400° F for 15 minutes until meat is browned.
- Drain any excess fat and pat dry with a paper towel if you wish.
- Apply your usual pizza sauce and toppings.
- Return to the oven and bake everything until cheese topping is bubbling.

Cheezza Base

- Beat 3 eggs and mix with a Fist of grated cheese.
- Spread the mixture over parchment paper on a baking sheet.
- Bake at 400° F for 15 minutes or until the cheese is golden.
- Remove and let cool until you're ready to add your normal pizza topping and sauce.
- Turn the heat up to 450° F and then bake everything for 5-10 minutes until golden brown.

Sugar in Coffee or Tea

I recommend going with a sugar substitute such as Splenda, Stevia or Equal. Splenda is my go-to sugar substitute and research has shown very little is retained in the body. The only caveat I have is don't have more than six packets in a day due to some research showing that it can lead to increased appetite.[75]

Soda

I'm not a fan of you having any soda regularly, but as this is the compromise section then let's get into it. Never, ever, ever go for a full-sugar soda. I don't care how much you love it, it's absolute junk to your body and terrible for your blood. I recommend switching to diet soda as a compromise. It is best still to limit a diet soda to one a day. And by one, I mean one 12oz can, not a Big-Gulp 36oz cup!

If you really want to make a healthy change, weaning yourself off diet soda is the way to go. Some people don't even care about soda, but they do enjoy the fizzy experience. If that's you, then I recommend going to a carbonated water, either plain or naturally sweetened.

Chocolate

If like me, you love chocolate, then giving it up can sometimes feel like the sky is falling in. The good news is chocolate is still okay, however, in slightly different portions and quality. I'm okay with my clients having one or two squares of 70%+ dark chocolate.

Dark chocolate isn't that sweet and contains more cocoa than milk chocolate. The other substitute for chocolate is coconut oil chocolate. This is a quick and easy treat that's quite filling and on plan. A sliver after a meal can satisfy that sweet craving.

- Mix 1 tsp. unsweetened cocoa powder with 1 heaped tbsp. of melted coconut oil together.
- Add some Stevia or Splenda for sweetness.
- Pour onto parchment paper and leave in the refrigerator for 30 minutes.

Milk & Milky Coffee

Coffee shops such as Starbucks are the new fast-food restaurant, and milky drinks are best avoided because of the amount of sugar in them. Having a Starbucks coffee or a glass of 2% or whole milk now and then is okay as your treat, but I'd rather you stick to water, or a milk alternative if you have a milk drink.

A common concern people have about milk alternatives is that it doesn't taste the same as cow's milk. However, like most things, after a while you can get used to the taste and may find you like alternative more.

If you're used to having milk or a milky coffee every day, it's important to break this habit. Change milk drinks to a once a week treat and no more. I tend to do this on a Friday or Monday. Either starting or ending my week with a treat coffee.

If it's coffee you like and not necessarily the milk, then switch to either an Americano, which is an espresso drink with added hot water. You can then have it black or with added heavy cream. I prefer to ask the Barista for heavy cream rather than having half & half.

When giving up milky coffee, most people report they initially miss the soothing, creaminess of a latte but soon adjust to an

Americano or plain coffee. And after a few weeks of abstinence you'll probably find milky coffee is way too sweet.

Candy Bars

On your way to cleansing your blood, you might have a day when you just want a candy bar. I know I do. On those days I recommend going with something like a Power Crunch bar as a treat. This bar contains a good amount of protein for a snack bar with not too many. Ideally, break the bar in two and have half a Power Crunch at a time. This makes a fun snack, but if you end up eating the whole thing, then that's still okay. I don't recommend having one every day, as breaking a candy habit is important, so go carefully with the Power Crunch.

Potato/Corn Chips

Many of my client's report getting home from work and devouring a bag of tortilla chips or a bag of Lays before dinner. This tends to be a habit response because they're tired and haven't eaten well during the day. Chips offer an enjoyable experience to the brain because of the crunch, flavor, and high carb content. Chips are also very easy to eat, and overdoing it is common.

If you've never looked at the nutrition label on a bag of chips, then the next section will help you see how easy it is to eat way too many carbs from chips. Also, chips are a common trigger food, and if this is one of your trigger foods, you know how deadly a bag can be.

One of my favorite alternatives to chips are cheese chips. These are just rounds of grated cheese cooked in an oven until crispy. I know that may sound weird, but this really is a healthier chip snack.

As cheese has zero carbs, and fats are very much part of this plan, you can have a fantastic crunchy, cheesy snack instead of high carb chips.

Cheese Chips

- Preheat oven to 375f
- On parchment paper or silicon sheet make small mounds of grated cheese with 1 tbsp. of cheddar or Mexican cheese mix.
- Bake for about 6 mins. but watch the last couple of minutes so you don't burn the cheese.
- Let cool and enjoy.
- Alternatively, you could use thin slices of Provolone, Edam or Halloumi.

Another alternative is pepperoni chips. If you're someone who loves pepperoni then you're in for a treat. Most stores carry pre-sliced pepperoni, and all you need to do is throw them on a kitchen towel and put them in the microwave for 1-3 minutes. The only problem is not eating too many of these because they are so delicious.

There are also many vegetables we can make as chips. The one I enjoy the most is baked butternut squash chips, sprinkled with some Parmesan cheese. It's really is easy to try out all kinds of different vegetables to see what hits that spot. I bake a lot of different vegetables to see what works for me.

Another option is to grab yourself a dehydrator. With this gadget you can make one of the most unlikely chips on the planet; blue cheese cucumber chips. Come on, be honest, never in your wildest dreams did you ever think cucumber could be a viable alternative to your chip fix, but they are. They come out crispy and flavorful from the dehydrator and contain next to no carbs, so you can go to town on these.

Maybe next time you have a party, try making several different types of chips and I bet you'll be amazed at how appreciative and curious your guests will be to have something other than standard chips.

Blue Cheese Cucumber Chips

- Cut the cucumber very thin. Using a mandolin is helpful.
- Lay cucumber in the dehydrator and place a knob of blue cheese (or any cheese) on each chip.
- Set the dehydrator to 135 F and leave for around 6 hours until crisp.

Spaghetti/Pasta/Noodles

Pasta is a classic favorite and I admit to having the occasional plate of spaghetti Bolognese or carbonara. However, the amount of carbs in a pasta dish should really scare you away from them as a regular food. The good news is the meat sauce part of spaghetti Bolognese or the cream and bacon of carbonara is a good choice.

A good alternative to spaghetti is zucchini noodles (also known as Zoodles). These are good and taste great when mixed in with the sauce. They can usually be found pre-made in many stores. Check out either the pre-cut vegetable section or the vegetarian section of your local store. Once you have your noodles, just added them to the meat sauce, stir in for about 3 minutes and serve.

Staying with vegetables, have you tried cabbage noodles? Nope, didn't think so. These aren't really noodles, but what I like to do is fry shredded cabbage in a pan, and then add my meat sauce over the top. Noodles are just a filler, which means you can add any vegetable you like to this dish as an alternative. I know it isn't the same, but it is still good.

My next alternative noodle are Shirataki noodles. These are noodles made from the konjac yam and once cooked it has a pleasant al dente texture. These can be used as spaghetti or even added to broth to make Ramen or Pho. These noodles are sometimes called Miracle Noodles and can be found in most stores in the vegetarian section. The only downside to these noodles is when you open the packet, they do smell, so make sure you rinse them for a couple of minutes before you begin the cooking process.

Lastly, there is the good old spaghetti squash alternative. This is another good vegetable that goes great with the meat sauce. However, this does take a little more work to prepare and can be somewhat watery. It might help to dry them on a paper towel before adding to your meat sauce.

Rice

A staple for many cultures. You may be wondering why rice is on the Whoa! List when many Asians report lower cases of diabetes and heart disease. This is more down to the fact they also eat very little sugar and processed foods unlike Western diets. I'm fine with you having about half a Fist of rice (equal to half a cup) now and then, but not regularly.

One alternative to rice which some people love is cauliflower rice. This is becoming more and more common in stores and packets can be found in the pre-sliced vegetable or vegetarian section. The other option is Miracle rice. This is made from a plant called Konnyaku which is just soluble fiber. This rice can also be found in most stores or online through Amazon and Walmart.

Potato

Having potato now and then is fine. A good portion of potato is about half a Fist which is usually about one small russet potato. If you're someone who eats a lot of potatoes, there are a few alternatives you might want to try. Kabocha squash has a fluffy sweet texture like sweet potato but it's very low in carbs. This is great when roasted just like a normal potato. You can also chop it up and make oven-baked fries, or in soups, salads and curries.

Jicama is another excellent alternative. You can eat these raw but they're more like a firm pear than a potato when eaten this way. You can make these into fries, and they do taste fantastic.

Cauliflower is a versatile vegetable, and as well as rice, you can use it to make cauliflower mash. Many clients say they like this a lot and are really surprised how good it tastes.

Lastly, you can always try Daikon radish. These aren't exactly a like-for-like alternative to potato, but they are low carb and they can be oven roasted and used where you might use potato. They're also great raw or steamed and have a texture like carrots.

Granola

Sometimes cereal just hits the mark in the morning, and even though I'm okay with a little oatmeal, having something a bit crunchier is fun. Store-bought granola in all its forms is not good because it's very high in sugar, especially with all the added honey, and dried fruit. Instead of buying your granola, making it at home. It's easy to do and you'll only need four ingredients.

This alternative granola is still going to be higher in carbs than say bacon and eggs, so a small portion is recommended. You can eat this granola with almond milk or add to your Greek yogurt.

Cinnamon Granola (6-8 servings)

- Take half cup of chopped or smashed walnuts, pecans, macadamia, and unsweetened coconut flakes and mix in a bowl.
- Stir in 2 tbsp. melted butter or melted coconut oil with 1-2 packets of Splenda and 1 tbsp. cinnamon.
- Grease a baking tin and spread a thin layer of granola.
- Bake at 350° F for 15-20 mins.
- Let cool and crumble into granola-sized chunks then store in an air-tight container.

Oatmeal

Now and then a small portion of oatmeal is fine for breakfast if it's still made in water and paired with some form of protein. But if you're looking to enjoy oatmeal more often, and still want to cut the carbs a little more, then try making your own oatmeal. It will still have carbs, mainly from seeds, but the addition of hemp seeds boosts the protein in this dish.

- Mix 1 heaped tbsp. of chia seeds, hemp seed, sunflower and flaxseed (whole not ground), into a cup of coconut milk or a mix of almond milk and heavy cream.
- Slowly bring to the boil and simmer until it thickens.
- Add a knob of butter or ghee to the top if you want to make it creamier.
- If you like it sweet, add a packet of Splenda or a pinch of salt for savory.
- Add cinnamon if you like.
- To make a batch, mix a cup of each seed and store.

BLT's and Other Sandwiches

If you're used to grabbing sandwiches for lunches, then you're going to need to expand your horizons and find alternatives. Luckily for you, I love making alternative sandwiches, and you can make almost any sandwich with lettuce leaves instead of bread or tortilla.

The outer shell of a sandwich is only there to hold the filling together, and I find romaine or butter lettuce leaves are perfect for this bread alternative. Just use the leaves the same way as you'd use bread and spread a little mayo or mustard on the leaf before adding your filling.

If you're used to tortilla wraps (which are still high in carbs), then just use the leaf in the same way. If you need more than one leaf to make the wrap larger, just overlay one over the other and roll. Simple.

Flour for Baking

For you bakers, finding alternatives to flour can be challenging because there isn't much that's as good as traditional flour. I know from my experiences of making bread alternatives that I can never get the mix as fluffy as traditional flour. However, flour alternatives can also be tasty in their own way. Usually, once we understand these alternatives are not going to be like-for-like we can enjoy them for what they are.

The best alternative flours are almond flour, coconut flour and tapioca flour. These are lower in carbs and still versatile, although they will be a little denser than all-purpose flour. I can make alternative muffins, pastry and bread and enjoy them. The main difference is they don't rise as well as tradition flour and can be a little dryer. If you find that is the case, add a generous helping of butter over it.

Almond Flour Raspberry Muffins

- Preheat oven to 325f
- Chop a cup of raspberries into bits.
- Line or grease a twelve-cup muffin tray.
- Mix together 3 eggs. 2 tbsp. melted coconut oil. 1 tbsp. lemon juice. 1 tbsp. vanilla extract. 2 tbsp. honey and 1-2 packets of Splenda. I mix this with a whisk and then put it in a blender to make it creamy.
- Mix 200g fine almond flour (I sieve mine first), 1/2 tsp. baking soda, and a small pinch of Himalayan salt.
- Add the wet mix to the flour and fold in the raspberries.
- Add to muffin tray.
- Bake for 20 to 25 mins. until the top is golden.
- Cool on a wire rack.

Understanding Nutrition Labels

Understanding nutrition labels is extremely important and if you haven't really paid much attention in the past, now is the time to learn a new skill. I think understanding labels is a fundamental step towards you taking responsibility for what you're eating because the information on the front of a package only tells you what the manufacturer wants you to think of their food. The truth of what you are eating is on the nutrition facts label.

Before you make any changes to your shopping list, I'd like to highlight a few more things about nutrition labels to make sure you make the best possible choices to help cleanse your blood. You will find manufacturers will use all kinds of tricks to make you think their food item is healthy with all kinds of claims on the front, but don't believe a word of it. Read the label before making up your mind.

Overall, pre-packaged foods are not going to be the most ideal choice for reversing your condition because they usually have a lot of added carbs and sugars. I understand sometimes we're short on time and need to make the best, quick food choices we can, and by understanding labels, you'll be in a better position to make informed choices on a few items that will work for you.

The only things on the label you need to concern yourself with are:
- The portion size of the food
- How much protein the food contains
- How many carbs and sugar the food contains
- How much fat the food contains
- How much fiber it might have, if any at all

Everything else on that label is extra information you don't need. You don't need to know the calories, as we don't count them. You don't need to know how many vitamins it contains. You don't need to know how much cholesterol is in the food, and you don't need to know the percentage of Daily Value the food represents.

If you have high blood pressure, then you might want to pay attention to the amount of sodium the food contains. As a guide, around 2300mg of sodium is one teaspoon of salt. If you don't have high blood pressure, you can be mindful of salt if you like, but you don't need to worry that much.

Here are a few 'label rules' I'd like you to focus on:

- Prioritize protein and fat over carbohydrates.
- Ideally, you'll be looking at around a 2:1 ratio of protein to carbs.
- Fiber is a good macro-nutrient to have in your diet. Try to choose a higher fiber choice if you're torn between two different foods which have similar protein, fat and carb content.

Example of a Single Portion Label

Nutrition Facts

Serving Size 1 (17g)
Servings Per Container 1

Amount Per Serving

Calories 90

	% Daily Value*
Total Fat 7.5g	12%
Saturated Fat 0.75g	4%
Trans Fat 0g	
Sodium 50mg	2%
Total Carbohydrate 4g	1%
Dietary Fiber 1.5g	6%
Sugars 1.5g	
Protein 3g	6%

*Percent Daily Values are based on a 2,000 calorie diet.

Here's a clear label from my favorite Barney's almond butter in a single portion pack. As you can see, this label clearly states the nutrition facts for a single serving packet (17g). The serving size is the first piece of information and the first thing I'd like you to notice on any label because this is where obfuscation happens when food manufacturers try to manipulate the label in their favor. A serving size doesn't always mean the whole packet, and we'll see an example of that in a moment.

On this single serving of almond butter, you can understand what is in this entire packet. You can have confidence that when you eat this almond butter, the amount of protein, fat and carbs you ingest is exactly what this packet claims.

This package also has a 1:1 ratio of protein to carbs, which for this type of food, I'm okay with. And the reason for that is this food is more of a fat-based snack, and less about the protein and carbs. This is essentially true with all nut-based foods. I'd have no problem with you eating this as a snack on its own or as a supplement to a protein meal to fill you up.

Example of a Multiple Serving Label

Nutrition Facts

8 servings per container
Serving size   15 (28g)

Amount Per Serving
Calories   **160**

	% Daily Value*
Total Fat 10g	13%
Saturated Fat 1.5g	8%
Trans Fat 0g	
Cholesterol 0mg	0%
Sodium 170mg	7%
Total Carbohydrate 15g	5%
Dietary Fiber 1g	4%
Total Sugars 1g	
Includes 0g Added Sugars	0%
Protein 2g	4%

Here's an example of a multiple serving label from a popular chip manufacturer. Because chips are typically high in carbohydrates, the label on this large packet of chips represents a *single serving*, even though there are multiple servings in a packet. If you look at the servings per container, you'll see they recommend this chip packet contains eight servings.

Technically there's nothing wrong with this label. They show the nutritional values, and all that's required of them by law, but what they don't tell you is how many calories, carbohydrates, fat, or protein there is in one entire packet, and I think that's wrong. If something contains more than one serving, there really ought to be a second label that shows what's in the packet you've brought. Otherwise, it can seem like the food manufacturers are trying to hide something.

Ask yourself, have you ever looked at the label on a large packet of chips or other food item, and then worked out what the carbs or calories are for the entire packet? Do you every portion out the servings as suggested? My guess is you don't, because I know I usually don't.

So, knowing that most of us won't portion out a bag of chips into eight servings, or even do the math of what's really in a full bag of chips, let's look at what a label for this entire packet would look like.

Nutrition Facts

1 servings per container

Serving size 1 (224g)

Amount Per Serving

Calories 1280

	% Daily Value*
Total Fat 80g	103%
Saturated Fat 12g	60%
Trans Fat 0g	
Cholesterol 0mg	0%
Sodium 1360mg	59%
Total Carbohydrate 120g	44%
Dietary Fiber 8g	29%
Total Sugars 8g	
Includes 0g Added Sugars	0%
Protein 16g	32%

If you picked up a large packet of chips and you saw this incredible label on the bag and you noticed how many carbohydrates, sodium and fat this packet contains, I pretty much guarantee you and most other people wouldn't buy it. And that's what food manufacturers count on.

Personally, I find this type of labeling very misleading and underhanded. In my view, the nutrition value should reflect the totality of the item you are buying and then let you, the consumer, decide how many servings suit your needs.

This servings size 'trick' happens on a lot of packaged foods, so be extra vigilant when you shop. Do pay attention to what a label is telling you, and soon enough you'll get the hang of what's a good and bad option.

More Package Information

Just because food manufacturers can't mess with the food label too much, that doesn't stop them from adding all kinds of hype, nonsense, and buzzwords onto the packaging to entice you into buying their product. As well as paying attention to the label, you might be interested to know some of the other tricks and claims manufacturers try and persuade you that their product is healthy.

The information below isn't going to help cleanse your blood but what I think this information will highlight is how manufacturers use terms to make you believe food is healthier than it is.

No Added Sugar

This is one of the sneakiest claims in this list and one which many people fall for. Just because there's no added sugar it doesn't mean it contains zero sugar. What this means is the product doesn't contain any *extra* sugar to the amount of sugar in the product already.

Basically, if a product contains fruit, wheat, grains, corn, milk or vegetables then it will have sugar in it. When you see this claim, be skeptical, because they're trying to fool you into thinking this is a low-sugar food and it probably isn't.

Sugar-Free

Just like no added sugar, sugar-free doesn't mean carbohydrate free, so you'll still need to pay attention to the label. A lot of sugar-free products are sweetened with sugar alcohols such as xylitol, erythritol or sorbitol which, in small doses (around 3g or less) I think is mostly fine. However, larger amounts can lead to bloating, gas and diarrhea. Remember, food sweetened with sugar-alcohols still have the same impact on blood glucose.[43]

Made with Real Fruit

Fruit is still sugar, so claiming something is made with real fruit means the product is going to contain sugar. The other thing with this type of claim is that manufacturers don't need to divulge how much fruit is used in the ingredients. It could be as little as 0.5% of the product but they can still claim it's made with real fruit. The reality is, a lot of foods which claim to be made with real fruit are going to be snack foods which you're best avoiding anyway.

All Natural or Natural

Just like Net Carbs, the term All Natural or Natural isn't regulated by the FDA. Unlike organic, there's no formal definition of what natural means. As long as it doesn't contain anything synthetic like artificial flavors or colors then they can call the food natural. But natural can still be somewhat processed.

However, just because a food claims to be All Natural and doesn't have synthetic additives it doesn't mean it won't contain other harmful ingredients such as high fructose corn syrup, genetically modified organisms (GMO), or growth hormones.

A lot of foods have thickeners or oils added to them which are natural but are not foods we would typically eat. For example, Snapple often advertises their drinks as All Natural and add the ingredient Ester Gum, which sounds innocuous enough. But Ester Gum's is an oil-soluble food additive whose full name is glycerol ester of wood rosin. And yes, you guessed it, it is made by combining the often-used sweet viscous liquid, glycerol (which is made from triglycerides), and the ester of wood rosin, AKA resin from pine trees. All Natural, maybe, All Natural without being processed first, no way.

Organic

This is one of the biggest buzzwords in food, and a consumer report has shown that on average, food prices for organic foods are increased by 47%.[53] You might see labels stating 'organic' on a product, but the trouble is, organic doesn't mean healthier or even better than the non-organic products.

Organic standards are set by the USDA's National Organic Program (NOP) and not the FDA, so unlike the unregulated term All Natural, to be classed as organic, 95% of the ingredients must meet the NOP standard and be grown without synthetic fertilizers or pesticides.

However, because only 95% needs to be organic, the other 5% can be non-organic or synthetic, including harmful things such as Carrageenan. In fact, there are 200 non-organic substances which can be included without influencing the organic status of a product.[54] And not only is organic food priced higher, there's very little evidence to support the claim that there are any health benefits to organic food over conventionally grown food.[55]

"But what about the environment? Organic is better for the soil, isn't it?" Thanks for the question, but the reality is, many non-synthetic pesticides are worse for the soil because more is used to be effective. Plus, organic pesticides still pose the same dangers as non-organic pesticides. Likewise, organic farming tends to need larger amounts of land than conventional farming to grow similar amounts of food; which means more machinery for harvesting, which leads to higher emissions and pollution.[56] Sadly, organic doesn't mean what we would like it to mean, and my advice, unless you really love the difference between organic and conventional, go with what suits your budget.

Made with Organic Ingredients

Another sneaky claim which doesn't enhance the nutrition value or quality of the food you're buying but can still bump the price. If something claims it's made with organic ingredients, only around 70% of that product needs to be organic. Just like organic food can have 5% non-organic ingredients in it, this can contain a whopping 30% of non-organic ingredients. So, everything I said about organic applies even more to this claim.

100% Organic

Just to confuse you more, there is a difference between organic produce, and 100% organic produce. As organic food is only 95% organic, with the other 5% potentially being a GMO, (even though it technically shouldn't be), or a product grown with synthetic pesticides. 100% organic means the produced ingredient must contain no additives or processing aids that are not organic. This means no synthetic pesticides were used, and the ingredients contain no GMO's.

Although it's nice to know the food we eat doesn't contain any synthetic pesticides, there's still little evidence to support significant benefits between organic food and conventional food. However, at least when something is 100% organic you have a better shot of getting a product that doesn't contain anything harmful, and this might sway me to go for 100% organic over conventional.

Non-GMO

Non-GMO stands for Non-Genetically Modified Organisms. This label is to counter the increasing amount of genetically modified food that's manufactured these days. A GMO product occurs when a gene is removed from an organism such as animal, bacterium, plant or even a virus, and is then added to a plant or animal to change its DNA. The idea behind this is to make the plant crop more abundant, resistant to weather or insects, or to make animals grow fatter to produce more milk. The trouble is, do we really want genetically modified food in our lives? A growing number of people are saying no, which is why you're seeing more Non-GMO labels popping up.

Here's a list of plants which are genetically modified in the USA:
- Alfalfa
- Arctic® Apples
- Canola
- Corn
- Cotton
- Papaya
- Innate® Potato
- Soybeans
- Sugar Beets
- Yellow Crookneck Squash
- Zucchini

One of the difficulties with GMO's is they may not always be in our food, but they are being fed to livestock which eventually will come into our food in diverse ways. In the US, cows are injected with a synthetic genetically-engineered hormone made from the E. Coli bacteria called Recombinant Bovine Growth Hormone (rBGH). This hormone makes cows produce around 10-15% more milk. The US is the only developed country to allow humans to drink milk from an rBGH-injected cow. In 27 other countries around the world, including the European Union, Japan, New Zealand, Argentina, Australia, and Canada, rBGH is banned because of the potential links to breast and gastrointestinal cancer.[57]

Due to concerns over GMO food, Non-GMO labels are gaining popularity, with the Non-GMO Project being the most recognized. However, the Non-GMO Project is a non-profit that has no ties to the

FDA or USDA's NOP, or any type of government regulation. Companies can join the Non-GMO Project, and the Project will verify that a member's food doesn't contain GMO's. What this verification doesn't account for is what's in the product, where the product came from, or under what conditions it was grown.

"So, why doesn't the FDA or USDA regulate GMO's?" Now that is a good question, but the FDA and USDA are clear they don't want to get involved with anything to do with genetically-modified foods.

The FDA has a policy of letting food producers volunteer whether their food is GMO or Non-GMO[58] and go as far as saying, and I quote from their website:

"The agency is not aware of any information showing that foods derived from genetically engineered plants, as a class, differ from other foods in any meaningful or uniform way. These foods also don't present different or greater safety concerns than their non-genetically engineered counterparts." [59]

Gluten Free

This is another label claim catching fire over the last few years, which is good and bad for people who have Celiac disease. If you don't know, Celiac disease is an autoimmune disorder which is caused by an intolerance to gluten which is the protein found in wheat, barley and rye. Basically, all the ingredients found in bread, pasta, and pretty much any product on the shelves of your local store. Celiac disease affects about 1% of the US population but many more people can have a condition called Non-Celiac Gluten Intolerance or Gluten Sensitivity.

How would you know if you're Gluten Sensitive? Well, the physical affects you might experience are bloating, cramping, constipation, diarrhea, and fatigue after eating something with wheat in it, and over time you might start experiencing chronic fatigue.

But, before you think of going gluten-free, I would say think again. Unless you have Celiac disease and don't have many other food choices, then there are several things to understand about what Gluten Free means.

Just like many of the other claims, this is a voluntary label which the FDA claims to oversee. Second, gluten-free doesn't mean the ingredients are organic or non-GMO's. In fact, many manufacturers will replace wheat for corn, because corn doesn't contain the protein which affects people with Celiac disease. However, we know corn is one the most genetically modified ingredients in the world. Plus, corn is very high in carbohydrates and that's going to affect your blood just as much as non-gluten food.

Just because something is gluten-free it can still contain wheat and grains because all the manufacturer does is remove the protein from the wheat and grains. Either way, the carbohydrate content in gluten-free food is still going to be high.

Studies have shown people with Celiac disease show an elevated risk of developing metabolic syndrome after one year on a gluten-free diet.[60]

Ultimately, unless you have Celiac disease, then gluten-free food is not any better for you and best left alone.

High Fiber or Good Source of Fiber

Fiber is important to a healthy diet, and many of my clients have been told to increase their fiber to help maintain bowel health, stay heart healthy, and reduce obesity. The problem with this advice is the way people are encouraged to get more fiber in their diet, rather than the message itself. Typically, the advice from a doctor is to eat more wheat bran, whole wheat, and grains, which for your condition is a bad idea because, yes you guessed, the high level of carbs in wheat and grains.

I do recommend making sure you get a lot of fiber in your diet, and the best way is to get fiber is eating more vegetables from the GO section. The traditional way of getting fiber through grains is only going to make you more insulin resistant.[61]

Free Range

Eggs can be an important source of your nutrition plan, so buying ethical eggs might be important to you. As you're probably becoming aware, what a label claims and what happens are often two different things and free range is no different.

Like most 'standards' on labels, there just aren't any. For the USDA's to consider an egg Free Range means the hens must have *access* to the outdoors. What this might conjure in your mind are images of chickens left to roam freely around pastures, scratching at dirt and having a pretty good time.

This is far from the truth. There are no requirements on the amount of outdoor space, they have access to. There are also no requirements on the duration of time they have access, or the quality of the outdoor space. The only access many hens have to the outdoors is from a small poop hole behind them. They do not have enough space to roam freely. Essentially, Free Range means next to nothing.

I recommend looking for Certified Humane® Free Range eggs, which is a certification from another voluntary non-profit, called Humane Farm Animal Care (HFAC) which does have set standards farmers need to adhere to in order to use that label. To qualify for the HFAC's Certified Humane® Free Range label, the hens must have 2sq. ft to roam in. And they need to be outdoors for at least six hours per day. Although the HFAC is still voluntary, I feel more comfortable with their approach to Free Range than the USDA's.

Doctor Recommended

This also means absolutely nothing. There are so many things wrong with this claim that if you see this on a package you need to just walk away. What this claim tells you is that in the entire world, out of millions of doctors, one doctor may have said they like the product or recommend it (or been paid to recommend it). Unless you know the doctor, who's recommending this product, and you trust their judgment and integrity, just ignore this claim completely.

Label Notes: Avoid Carrageenan

While we're looking at labels, you won't find the name Carrageenan on the box, but you will find it on the ingredients list. I want to add it here as I feel this ingredient is something to make sure is not added into any food or drinks you have. This additive contains no nutritional value and is used to thicken food. However, the main problem with Carrageenan is that it's been linked to inflammation in the body.

Research on mice shows ingesting low levels of Carrageenan over 18 days lead them to develop glucose intolerance and impaired insulin action. Both eventually leading to diabetes. This may not do the same in humans, but again it might. If in doubt, I advise avoiding any product containing Carrageenan.[63,64,65,66]

PART FOUR:

YOUR BLOOD

"Good health and good sense are two of life's greatest blessings."
- Publilius Syrus

Understanding Your Blood

You may have come to this book with little to no idea about diabetes, prediabetes, and metabolic syndrome, and that's okay. What I hope to do over these pages is help you understand a little more about what is going on in your body, what your condition is, and how it affects your entire system. I also want to demystify your lab results and help you understand what all the numbers and names mean so you can read a report with confidence. Understanding what is happening in your blood and having the skill to read your blood results will enable you to have informed conversations with your doctor about your condition.

If you've lived with your condition for a while, you may think you understand your problem well. But you might be surprised with what is really happening inside you, because much of what the media or even many doctors might tell you about your blood condition, is not always helpful and often misleading. It might be useful to you to read through this section, even if you think you know what's going on and I will try and help you understand a complex subject in a simple way.

As you know, my training is as a psychotherapist and I am in no way an endocrinologist, and I don't pretend to be a doctor. However, all the information I have written here is based on my experience of working with people like you, alongside doctors who specialize in this field. Plus, everything I write in this section is backed-up by a whole lot of current research. For your peace of mind, if the information I tell you isn't factual and backed by research, it's not in this book.

Diabetes

The truth is, even now, we still don't know the entire reason for diabetes, but we do understand a lot more about the condition than we used to. Historically, being diabetic meant your body couldn't maintain healthy blood sugar levels (sugar=glucose, remember), but this isn't exactly true. Having high blood sugar is absolutely a symptom and does cause you to be sick. However, the main reason you have diabetes is because of a hormone problem, namely the hormone insulin. We'll go into insulin a lot more over the coming pages, but essentially its main function is to deliver sugar energy to cells in your body, such as your muscles.

Because insulin works in conjunction with blood sugar, you either you have too much insulin pumping around your body or your body doesn't produce enough insulin. For now, all you need to know is blood sugar and insulin are a little like two countries in an arms race - the more your blood sugar goes up, the more insulin you produce, and the more insulin you produce the more your blood sugar goes up. Soon your body stops functioning properly and this state is called *insulin resistant*.

We'll talk more about this later, but for me, one of the reasons people stay diabetic or even pre-diabetic for as long as they do, is because of the unhelpful tendency to just focus on blood sugar as the problem. I believe more people would get better help if they recognized this condition as hormone imbalance.

Diabetes Mellitus Type-1

- Used to be called juvenile-onset or insulin-dependent diabetes.
- Usually develops in children and teenagers but can develop at any age.
- This condition is caused by the body attacking its own pancreas, which means the body can't produce insulin.

- With this condition, the person will be on insulin from injections or fitted with an insulin pump. This pump delivers insulin into the body automatically throughout the day.
- Since 2016, a new type of artificial pancreas or closed-loop delivery system has been used. This device is implanted into the body and monitors glucose levels through the day, delivering the correct amount of insulin when needed.
- Typically, someone with Type-1 will be on lifelong insulin therapy.

Diabetes Mellitus Type-2

- Used to be called adult-onset or non-insulin dependent diabetes.
- It can develop at any age.
- About 90% of people diagnosed with diabetes will have Type-2.
- Most people don't realize they have Type-2 and can have it years until they're diagnosed following a blood test.
- With Type-2, the pancreas either doesn't produce enough insulin to remove sugar from the blood, which is called insulin deficient; or it can't produce enough because the cells in the body are insulin resistant.
- Many people with Type-2 will be given oral medication to control their blood sugar or they'll inject insulin to increase the amount of insulin the body can use.
- Type-2 diabetes is reversible with healthy lifestyle changes and doesn't need to be a lifelong condition.

Gestational Diabetes

- This happens during pregnancy when a woman's blood sugar levels rise due to the fetus needing more glucose to help it grow.
- Hormone changes during pregnancy make insulin less effective, leading to insulin resistance. If the woman's body cannot produce

enough insulin to overcome this resistance, then her blood glucose level becomes abnormally high.
- Other factors which increase the potential risk of getting gestational diabetes are being overweight, and if the mother has a history of diabetes in the family.[1]
- Blood glucose levels tend to return to normal after childbirth, but there is a greater risk of developing Type-2 later in life, so extra care is needed.

Prediabetes

- Prediabetes means your blood sugar levels are high but not quite high enough to be in the diabetic range.
- There are nearly three times as many people in the US who have prediabetes than diabetes, but this figure is most likely significantly higher as most people don't realize they have prediabetes, as there are very few obvious signs or symptoms.
- Most people with prediabetes will develop diabetes over the next five years.

Metabolic Syndrome

- This condition occurs when you're diagnosed as having a cluster of conditions, or risk factors.
- These risk factors are high blood sugar, high triglycerides, low HDL cholesterol, high blood pressure, and excessive fat around the belly.
- Metabolic syndrome is heavily under-diagnosed, as most people don't realize they have metabolic syndrome as there are no visible signs except an excessive amount of fat around the belly.
- People with metabolic syndrome are just as at risk of health-related problems like heart disease or stroke as somebody with diabetes. It's no lesser a condition.

- Metabolic syndrome risk factors are present in four of the top ten killing diseases in the US.
- The way to reverse metabolic syndrome is much the same as reversing diabetes and prediabetes with lifestyle changes.

The Path to Diabetes

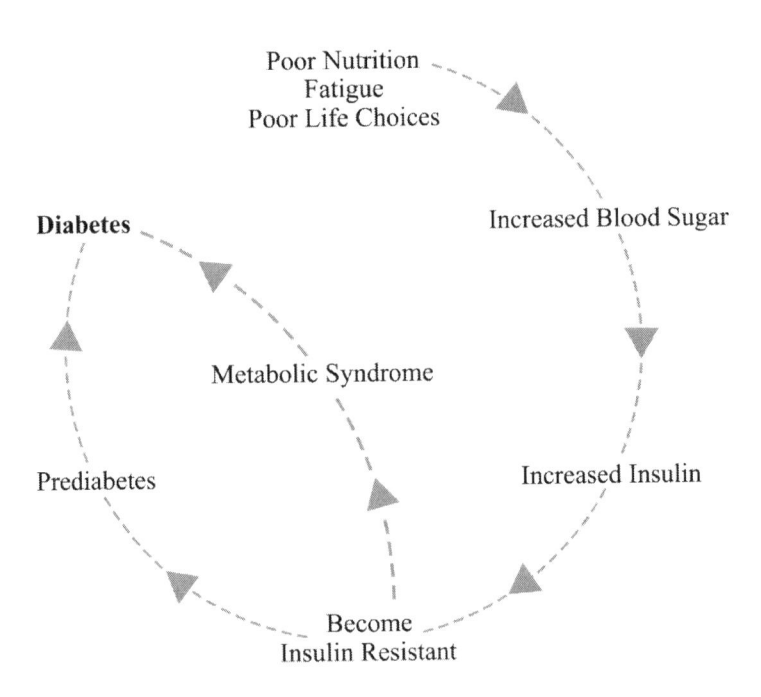

```
              Poor Nutrition
                 Fatigue
              Poor Life Choices

  Diabetes                         Increased Blood Sugar


             Metabolic Syndrome

  Prediabetes                      Increased Insulin


                    Become
                Insulin Resistant
```

The image above shows a typical path to having diabetes and for many this can take years. Yet, with each stop on the cycle you are increasing your chances of chronic disease. I've seen this play out in different ways and I know without changing some aspects of lifestyle choices, at the very least you'll become insulin resistant, and at worst, fully diabetic.

One thing to note is you don't have to have metabolic syndrome to end up with diabetes. The perception is usually 'fat and lazy' people have diabetes and metabolic syndrome, but this is untrue. Even thin, active, athletic people can end up with diabetes. They might not show signs of excess body fat around their mid-section or have high blood pressure or any of the other risk factors associated with metabolic syndrome, but they still end up diagnosed with diabetes. This is because these blood conditions are not solely driven by the food we eat. The path to diabetes can come from a multitude of unhealthy lifestyle choices.

In America alone diabetes and prediabetes are becoming a major problem with just under 50% of the population, over 120 million people, diagnosed with these conditions.[3] Just think about that for a moment. 120 million people sick and growing sicker. But the most incredible thing about that number is that it hardly covers the rest of the population who are highly likely to be insulin resistant and, on the way, to becoming diabetic if nothing in their lifestyle is changed.

If you don't think diabetes, prediabetes or metabolic syndrome are big issues, my hope is that you'll readjust your thinking after reading this book. Diabetes is an incredibly serious and life-altering condition, that deserves our full attention. And what a lot of people don't realize is how diabetes does kill people. It's what I call a slow killer, because it may not kill you fast like cancer, but in time, it can kill you.

Diabetes also affects you in physical ways which rob you of your health and can make living a productive life extremely difficult.

Physical Damage Due to Long-Term Diabetes

- Damage to the large blood vessels in the heart, brain, and legs (macrovascular complications).
- Retinopathy – blood vessels in the eye become damaged, which affects vision.
- Macular edema – when the eye's blood vessels are damaged and swelling occurs leading to blurred vision.
- Cataracts – the eye lens becomes cloudy, distorted, and sensitive to light.

- Glaucoma – fluid build-up in the eye becomes unhealthy and damaging.
- Neuropathy (nerve damage) in your hands, feet, legs, stomach, chest, and nerves controlling the organs.
- Constantly sore feet, including painful foot ulcers.
- Lack of feeling in the feet which can lead to damage that you are unaware of.
- Reduced healing in limbs from minor damage can become severe enough to lead to amputation.
- Clawed toes.
- Very dry skin, especially on the feet.
- Increased risk of tooth decay and gum disease.
- Reduced immune system.
- Increased risk of thyroid disease – overactive or underactive thyroid.
- Erectile dysfunction from nerve damage or reduced blood flow to the penis.
- Diabetic coma – ketoacidosis coma, hyperosmolar coma or hypoglycemic coma.

Not good, right? And all this can be avoided with the right guidance and a few lifestyle changes. I've seen what diabetes did to my father and I know he didn't just wake up one day with the condition. He, like everyone else, started off from a healthy place, and then through environmental factors and poor lifestyle choices he became insulin resistant which lead to a heart attack. Before dying several years later, he suffered with nearly all the above physical damage due to his unchecked diabetes. And believe me when I say, you really don't want to go out that way.

Metabolic Syndrome

If we look at metabolic syndrome (formerly known as Syndrome X), this condition really is a bigger deal than it may sound. Although diabetes hogs most of the limelight, in many ways metabolic syndrome is more of a health risk than diabetes and prediabetes because it doesn't just have one risk factor associated with it (high blood sugar), it has several risk factors. You are also five times more likely to have diabetes in the next five years if things don't change. Metabolic syndrome is a clear steppingstone to diabetes.[4]

Metabolic syndrome is quickly becoming one of the major medical and public health problems facing the United States, with one in three people being diagnosed with this condition.[5] Unlike diabetes and prediabetes, there isn't just one thing we point to in metabolic syndrome to conclude you have the condition. Instead, these collection of risk factors increase your chances of developing other physical illnesses like heart disease, or stroke.

Unlike diabetes and prediabetes, high fasting blood glucose isn't always present in metabolic syndrome. My clients often have a blood glucose levels in a normal range - 90mg/dL - which is way below a risk factor. What I typically start to see in somebody with metabolic syndrome is a steady increase in fat around the belly area. This is often called central, or visceral obesity. Now, fat gain isn't always typical, and you might not be at that stage yourself, but research shows a gain in fat is a high predictor of metabolic syndrome. In fact, only 5% of people with metabolic syndrome are considered normal weight, while 22% are overweight and 60% of individuals are classified as obese.[6]

Later in this chapter I'll explain more about blood tests and lab results but here are the five risk factors to be diagnosed with metabolic syndrome.

Five Risk Factors of Metabolic Syndrome:

- A waist circumference over 35" for women, and 40" for men.
- High triglycerides greater than 150mg/dL (these are a type of fat found in the blood).
- Low HDL cholesterol 40mg/dL for men, 50mg/dL for women (one function of HDL is to remove cholesterol from your arteries).
- High blood pressure greater than 130/85mmHg (this is the reading of blood pumping against your arteries).
- High fasting glucose levels of 100mg/dL or greater.

Each of these factors is tied to insulin resistance: the increase in belly fat, the increase in triglycerides, and increase in high blood pressure.[7] The good news is if we can attack insulin resistance and make your body more insulin available, then we'll be able to help you lose body fat and reverse these conditions, regardless of your starting blood sugar levels.[8,9]

Like diabetes and prediabetes, there is often a malaise around metabolic syndrome. I see a lack of urgency to rectify the problem because it doesn't seem life threatening, but there is no doubt, we are experiencing a massive rise in the rates of obesity, diabetes, prediabetes and metabolic syndrome in the US and the rest of the world.

I want to be clear about this, metabolic syndrome may not sound scary, but it can be just as much of a killer as diabetes. Just so you are aware, these following problems are things you might face if metabolic syndrome isn't reversed.

Potential Metabolic Syndrome Health Problems

- Diabetes
- Heart Disease
- Nonalcoholic fatty liver disease

- Stroke
- Hormone imbalance in women like polycystic ovarian syndrome (PCOS which is a condition of growing small cysts in the ovaries)
- Kidney disease
- Obstructive Sleep Apnea (OSA)
- Dementia

What is Insulin?

I've mentioned insulin resistance a few times and before we tackle how to reverse insulin resistance, it might help to know what insulin really does.

Basically, when we eat food, this food is broken down in the gut, and the beta cells in the pancreas (which is like a six-inch long sausage that sits just off-center in your abdomen, just behind your stomach, and below the liver) will secrete a protein hormone called insulin which regulates how glucose is absorbed into the body's cells. This glucose is then used as energy. The amount of insulin released depends on the type of food that it's dealing with. We typically get energy from three various sources: carbohydrates, protein, and fats. Each has a different effect on the body, and each will affect insulin release differently.

For example, from a neutral blood sugar baseline (this might be blood sugar which is measured on an empty stomach), when we eat carbohydrates our insulin levels increase ten times higher than the baseline. If we compare that to fat and protein, these two macronutrients only increase insulin release twofold from the baseline.[2] What this means is that if we eat something carbohydrate heavy like a bagel or a high sugar drink like Coca-Cola, it causes our blood glucose to rise higher and faster, which means our pancreas will need to release a lot more insulin to deal with the heightened sugar in the blood. This doesn't happen if we eat fats, like a piece of cheese, for example, or protein, such as chicken.

Because insulin is a powerful regulator of metabolism and its job is to signal either energy consumption in the cells or drive energy storage when there's too much glucose, it's important that we do all we can to help this hormone do its job properly. And one of the easiest things we can do is eat better-balanced meals of protein, fats, and carbohydrate. When we focus more on using protein and fats as our main sources of food, our body has an excellent system to deal with the incoming slow-release energy and produces less insulin.

However, problems start to arise when we ingest more carbs and sugar than anything else. Because the body can only use or store so much energy in our muscles and liver, if we have any excess glucose energy floating around it needs to be cleaned out of the blood and stored elsewhere. The body does this by storing extra glucose energy as body fat. That's right, if you're storing more body fat than you used to, then it could be a sign you have too much glucose and insulin in your body and you might already be insulin resistant.

Not only does excess glucose lead to more fat storage, insulin also begins to inhibit that fat from being broken down, which makes it even harder for excess fat to leave the body. This is partly why losing weight can be hard for people who have become insulin resistant.

Becoming Insulin Resistant

Insulin resistance occurs over time and you really won't notice it's happening. You see, when your blood sugar levels are healthy, your body releases an appropriate amount of insulin to deal with the amount of sugar in your blood. This is the balance we want. But things go wrong and you continuously have more and more glucose entering your system, more insulin needs to deal with it. In time, our body becomes overwhelmed by the glucose onslaught and becomes less able to manage your blood sugar.

This generally happens because the cells which normally accept glucose for energy, are getting full and put up a *'closed'* sign. What this means is your cells are starting to become *resistant* to the insulin hormone which delivers the glucose to your cells.

How this works is when insulin arrives at a cell that is now *closed* what the insulin tries to do is force the glucose into that cell. It does this by making the pancreas pump more and more insulin into your bloodstream to deal with your mounting blood sugar and resistant cells (or you do this through add insulin through an insulin injection). This forcing of the blood sugar into your cells comes at a cost because over time, not only are your cells becoming resistant to insulin, but by not letting the glucose energy into your cells, more and more sugar is saturating your blood. In time high quantities of sugar in your blood becomes toxic to you. This really is a bad combination of things to start going wrong.

A metaphor I often use to explain this scenario is to imagine every day your mailman or woman arrives to deliver one or two letters to your mailbox. On any given day, this isn't a problem. However, imagine you start getting more mail (maybe you have a fan club because you're so gorgeous - oh yes you are). Your mailman turns up with two whole bags of mail and he starts stuffing the mail into your box. It might be a tight squeeze, but the mail goes in, but there's no room for anything more.

Now imagine the next day the same mailman turns up again with three bags of mail this time. He tries to stuff the mail into your box, but it won't go. Instead of stopping because there's no room. He calls five more mailpersons to help him push the mail into your mailbox. They get a few extra letters in, but they still have three bags left over, and they place these on your lawn.

The next day, not only do you have three bags on your lawn, but now you have three more bags turn-up. This time ten mailpersons come to help push the mail into your box. This goes on and on. Soon your mailbox breaks, plus you have a hundred sacks of mail on your lawn and an army of USPS workers standing around your front lawn.

Your whole house is overwhelmed by mail. Mail trucks are causing congestion in your road. But you know what's worse, the next day it comes again. Just because the mailbox is full, and your lawn is covered in hundreds of bags of mail and there are more mail people in one place than the world has ever seen, you're still getting multiple deliveries a day and the problem is getting worse. Doesn't that sound dysfunctional? Well, that is what is going on inside you, out of sight.

This cycle of increased glucose and insulin can go on for years without you seeing much physical change. Eventually, that will change. Insulin resistance is the starting point of when things go wrong, which is why it's ultimately important that you not only reduce your blood sugar levels, but your focus is on helping your cells become more *insulin sensitive*. What this means is you need to help your system get back into balance by helping your cells more amenable to accepting glucose. I talk about how to do this in the Five Pillars to Good Health section

The other issue you may have if you're insulin resistant is after a while it doesn't take a lot of carbohydrates to overwhelm the system. Even the smallest amount of carbs can have a detrimental effect on your weight and blood sugar. This is why a lot of people who are very overweight don't need to eat many carbs to keep gaining body fat, and their blood sugar levels keep rising. To somebody who's insulin resistant, even a small amount of carbohydrates and sugar will be like eating a lot.

Signs You Might Have an Insulin Problem

- Your waist starts to get bigger and will feel quite hard to the touch
- You might start craving high sugar/carbohydrate foods like soda, cookies, ice cream, pizza, and chips.
- You might start getting acne or large pores on your face and experiencing greasy skin.
- You may start to see more skin tags appear on your body.
- You might experience hair loss around the front and sides of your head.

- You might see some dark, crinkly-looking skin around your neck, groin or armpits; this is called Acanthosis Nigricans.
- You might even look a bit puffy and experience water retention/swelling in your joints, such as ankles or fingers.
- You may be experiencing more headaches, dizziness and blurred vision than normal.

These signs are a good indicator that you are insulin resistant and are on the way to having metabolic syndrome and/or diabetes or prediabetes if you haven't already been diagnosed.

What's Happening to Your Hormones?

What I hope you're beginning to understand from this book is diabetes, prediabetes, and metabolic syndrome are conditions caused by a hormone imbalance in our body. However, it's not just the hormone insulin that isn't working as it should, but several other hormones are falling out of balance. Our intricate hormone stability is there to make sure our body works efficiently and survives but when our hormones stop doing their assigned tasks, we will get sick.

Most people have heard of the hormones testosterone and estrogen, but there are other hormones working inside our body to keep us healthy. For a moment, I'd like to encourage you to take a minute to think about what really goes into making you human. I'd encourage you to see yourself as more than a just a body that thinks. Because inside your skin suit, there's an intricate, and extremely complex system working hard that we're mostly unaware of.

There are many problems associated with diabetes, prediabetes and metabolic syndrome, but the primary focus for most doctors is controlling high blood sugar, often giving medication to control it if necessary.

The problem with the sole focus being on blood sugar alone is that it's only one aspect of the problem, and not necessarily the most important. This is because, in my opinion, general physicians aren't in the habit of checking how well your insulin levels or other hormones are working, and whether they are contributing to your high blood sugar, high triglycerides or other risk factors.

It's easier to track blood sugar than understand how well your hormones are working (and cheaper). But without good hormonal balance it doesn't really matter how your blood sugar is doing, because your internal system is fighting itself and leading you to become sicker and sicker.

Hormones Out of Balance Due to Insulin Resistance

I know I keep going on about hormones, and I'm sure you get the picture, but just to drive home my point, I want to introduce you to four other hormones which become dysfunctional when you have diabetes, prediabetes, and metabolic syndrome, and they are rarely, if ever, talked about.

Sex Hormone–Binding Globulin (SHBG)

You'd be forgiven for not knowing much about the SHBG hormone regarding your condition because our old friend insulin tends to get most of the limelight. SHBG is a glycoprotein produced in the liver and binds to three sex hormones found in men and women: testosterone, estrogen and dihydrotestosterone (DHT). And what SHBG does is controls the amount of these hormones your body can use.

I'm sure you know how important testosterone and estrogen are for overall good health in men and women, but did you know one complication that can arise when SHBG levels are low? Insulin resistance, metabolic syndrome diabetes and gestational diabetes.[10,11]

Emerging research shows SHBG mediates cell-surface signaling and cellular delivery, which is part of the problem we have when someone is insulin resistance. Remember the '*closed*' sign on your cells? This means your cells just won't take the insulin-laden glucose for energy.[12]

And because SHBG levels are low, and you are insulin resistant, your pancreas is pumping more insulin into your body to compensate.

From here another vicious cycle continues as more insulin means your SHBG hormone levels drop even lower leading to impaired glucose control.[13,14] And impaired glucose control means higher blood sugar. Get the picture?

What this information is telling us is you might have your blood condition not because your diet is bad or anything like that, but because your sex hormones are not working properly.

If you haven't had your SHBG levels checked by your doctor, now might be the time to get it checked. Because if your SHBG levels are low, then cleansing your blood could be harder to do without this hormone functioning properly.

Glucagon

As insulin has the important task of getting glucose out of our blood, there's also another hormone whose job it is to be the antithesis of insulin. Its job is to raise our glucose levels when they become too low.

The protein hormone, glucagon, exists in the liver and can be thought of as being the backup energy source for the body.[15]

The best analogy I can give you is to imagine your body is like a hybrid car. The car's main source of fuel comes from petroleum but there are times of lower energy need, and that's when the battery can take over running the car. Just like petroleum, food is our main fuel and after eating, our blood sugar is at its highest and most plentiful, giving us enough fuel for our energy needs. This is when insulin is released to deliver this fuel to the cells where it's needed.

Now, when we don't eat, between meals or when we sleep, our primary fuel source is missing and our blood sugar drops, therefore our body needs to create its own fuel. Just like the hybrid car, when the demand for fuel is lower and the battery takes over, so does glucagon.

In these quiet periods, glucagon is released from the pancreas and tells the liver to release stored glucose to keep the system ticking over while no food-fuel is coming in. It is a very clever feedback system that makes sure we always have enough glucose energy to keep us going, especially in our brain which needs about 25% of our energy requirements.

When healthy, this system works flawlessly. However, when we become insulin resistant and our body is pumping more and more insulin into our bloodstream, this glucagon hormone stops doing what it's supposed to do and starts to do the opposite.[16] Instead of the pancreas shutting off glucagon when insulin triggers it to because there's an abundance of glucose in the blood, the pancreas for some reason thinks our blood sugar is low and switches the glucagon on. By doing this our blood sugar rises even higher and for a longer period.

What this means is your glucose not only stays high through the meal when it is normally high, but also between meals and throughout the day - it just doesn't drop. This is clearly not good for your blood condition. New research is looking into how to reduce glucagon influence on blood sugar, which brings us to our next important hormone.

Ghrelin

Ghrelin is a hormone which is secreted in the gut when it registers it's empty and needs more food-fuel. When this happens, ghrelin sends a signal through your bloodstream to the hypothalamus in your brain, which then tells you to go eat some food.[17] This is another cool hormone, but this hormone doesn't just let you know you're hungry. Oh no, new research shows us it does a lot more.

Ghrelin is also responsible for signaling to the body that it needs to decrease energy thermogenesis and oxidation in your fat cells. What this essentially means is if you go too long without eating, your body will stop burning fat just in case of starvation, and what makes this really important for people with metabolic syndrome, or if you are trying to generally lose weight, is that when you cut back on eating because you think it might help you lose weight, or if you're not eating enough because you are on some type of restrictive diet, then your ghrelin hormone will tell your body to stop burning fat. Because of this, you'll have this paradox of eating less to lose weight, but your body's resisting your efforts by releasing less fat because it fears starving. Which is why most people who follow fad diets will begin to stop losing weight after 4-6lbs and typically begin to gain that weight back.

This idea of starvation control may not make much sense in our food-abundant society, but our internal system has developed over thousands of years and it doesn't care that you have a grocery store down the road full of food.

Not only is ghrelin responsible for reducing energy expenditure and storing fat but research has shown ghrelin to be a key regulator of insulin resistance and diabetes, independent of food intake. Ghrelin is an important player in glucose stability through Gluconeogenesis and Glycogenolysis in the liver - or in plain English, regulation of blood sugar by regulating the release of glucose in the liver from our old friend glucagon.[18, 19, 20, 21]

This is important because it seems one of ghrelin's tasks is to increase glucagon release in the liver [22], which as we've covered above, becomes somewhat dysfunctional when we become insulin resistant.[23] Ah, the hormone imbalance links are getting longer!

The main problem we face with ghrelin is our conditions of diabetes, prediabetes and metabolic syndrome all inhibit ghrelin from functioning properly, and when ghrelin doesn't work effectively, we may find that we're hungry more often, which also plays a role in how leptin hormone (more info below) also functions.

When ghrelin is not working correctly, and we're in a constant state of hunger, usually our brain will encourage us to choose more carb/sugar heavy foods because it knows it can get the fastest energy from those types of food. Plus, when ghrelin isn't working well, it's not able to regulate other hormones which affect our blood sugar, namely our stress hormone epinephrine, which elevates our blood sugar even more.[24]

Another concerning inhibitor of ghrelin is the drug Metformin. This highly prescribed drug is often the first drug given to somebody with high blood sugar and its main job is to help reduce blood sugar.

But even though it does decrease blood sugar a little for some people, it generally doesn't decrease it enough to justify its continued use. In some ways, Metformin acts more like a weight loss drug because it can have an impact on suppressing appetite. The idea being, the less you eat, the fewer carbs you probably ingest, which leads to your blood sugar going down.[25]

Sadly, this drug facilitates even more ghrelin hormone dysfunction, and clearly, if ghrelin is not functioning properly, then it will have a negative effect on your blood sugar and insulin regulation. This seemingly conflicting cycle seems to put you into an unsatisfactory situation where this drug really isn't an effective way to manage high blood sugar.

Leptin

Leptin is often referred to as the 'fullness hormone'. In the short term, its job is to let the body know that you've eaten enough food to maintain your body fat mass. When it recognizes this mass has been maintained, it sends another signal to your hypothalamus to tell you to stop eating. It's the yang to ghrelin yin.

In the long-term, it's responsible for maintaining a healthy body weight by organizing the storing and losing of fat mass and like all the hormones we're looking at, when things are working right, they do a fantastic job, but when things start to go wrong, they really go wrong.

Leptin is an under-reported reason why your blood sugar and body fat are rising and is often overlooked as a source of your condition and conversely, overlooked to reverse it.

How can that be? Well, leptin works with insulin in this feedback loop - leptin tells your brain how much to eat, so you eat. The food is then turned into glucose, and insulin is released to transport the energy to your cells. When there's excess sugar it stores the energy away in fat cells which leptin also regulates. It does this because leptin is produced in fat, therefore the more fat you store, the more leptin you produce.[26] This rise in fat and leptin production eventually produces a condition called Leptin Resistant.[27]

Strangely, you'd think the more leptin hormone being produced would signal to the brain to stop eating instead of eating more. However, this is the problem with a rise in leptin, just as it is with insulin - the more this hormone saturates your blood the more your brain becomes deaf to its signals and you end up becoming chronically hungry. Which means your brain, once again tells you that you're chronically hungry. And like ghrelin dysfunction, you overeat, especially quick-energy foods like pizza, chips, bread, and candy which feeds back into your body releasing more insulin to deal with it. Which then breaks your liver hormone glucagon and your blood sugar skyrockets. Boom! The system fails and works against you, rather than for you.

What this all means is leptin isn't really a 'fullness hormone' to prevent you gaining body fat, it's actually part of the evolutionary starvation function to make sure your brain knows to store more fat during times of energy deficiency. And because your insulin resistance seems to break the healthy functioning of other hormones, your starvation signal is stuck in the *'on'* position to the detriment of your overall health.[28]

It seems like a strange paradox the more we eat, the more our hormones do the opposite of what they are supposed to do. But there is a clue in nature to why this might be, and we see this in certain animals who hibernate during the winter, like bears for example.

In the autumn months, you'll often see bears eating a lot more food to fatten up, so they can sleep away the winter. What happens is bears aim to eat more sugar, because it's a quick way to create fat, which is why they get their main source of sugar from fructose in berries.

In the months before winter, their appetite mechanism is switched off and they go into a state called Polyphagia, which leads to excessive hunger - very similar to what happens when our hormones stop functioning properly.

We see this in our choices of food when we have diabetes, prediabetes, and metabolic syndrome. We gravitate more towards carbohydrates, and the more sugar or fruit we eat, the more we could be telling our body that we are going into hibernation mode and need to store more fat. The problem is, unlike bears, we don't hibernate, and we don't go into a long fasting state where we burn off that fat mass for fuel. Instead, we become sick.

In time, we see our cells become desensitized to insulin, ghrelin, and leptin by overexposure to these hormones. The other unfortunate problem we now face is our blood sugar is rising out of control, and the treatment offered to lower blood sugar is compounding the problem.

Metformin, insulin injections, and restrictive diets all play a role in worsening our condition rather than offering a real remedy for good health because they negatively influence an already out-of-balance hormone system.

I hope what you've read so far about the dysfunction of your hormones is helping you see that diabetes, prediabetes, and metabolic syndrome are more complex than just having too much sugar in your blood. They are, in fact, a major result of your body circulating far too much insulin, which results in the shutting off the checks and balances which keep your hormones and body functioning well.

It really is a vicious cycle, and probably exhausting to read - and exhausting to your body!

Your Blood Work

Okay, so let's get down to the personal stuff and look at your blood work and what all the jargon and numbers mean. I've been working with doctors for a long time, and I'm amazed at how much knowledge they have but how little they communicate about what's really going on with us non-medical people. Over the years, I've explained to my client's what's going on with their blood work just as I am with you. And I do this mainly because their doctor didn't really go into more detail other than something was good, or bad. But what does that mean? Well, read on my curious friend, all will be revealed.

Your Lab Work

When you get a copy of your blood work, it will usually be called a Lipid Panel. Lipid means fat and what this test is generally looking for is how your cholesterol levels are doing. You might also have other tests included in a Lipid Panel depending on what your doctor is testing for.

The other two tests which are important for us to look at and understand are the Glucose test and the Hemoglobin A1c test. If your glucose levels have shown to be high, or your doctor has suspicions of new onset diabetes, you doctor is likely to check both glucose and A1c tests to confirm if you are diabetic.

In the first blood test example below, I've included glucose and A1c on the same test, but it isn't shown this way in regular lab reports (this is just for demonstration purposes). All the other test examples show either a Glucose or A1c test, but not both.

Just to note, your paperwork may not look like the versions I use for these examples.

Fasting Lipid Panel Blood Test With Added Glucose & A1c

Lipid Panel	Result	Flag	Reference Range
CHOLESTEROL, TOTAL	166		125-200 mg/dL
HDL CHOLESTEROL	36	LOW	> OR = 46 mg/dL
TRIGLYCERIDES	107		< 150 mg/dL
LDL-CHOLESTEROL	109		< 130 mg/dL (calc)
CHOL/HDLC RATIO	4.6		< OR = 5.0 mg/dL (calc)
NON HDL CHOLESTEROL	130		mg/dL (calc)

Target for non-HDL cholesterol is 30 mg/dL higher than LDL cholesterol target.

| GLUCOSE | 97 | | 65 - 99 mg/dL |

Hemoglobin A1c with eAG

| HEMOGLOBIN A1C | 5.5 | | <5.7% of total Hgb |

For the purpose of screening for the presence of diabetes
<5.7% Consistent with the absence of diabetes
5.7-6.4% Consistent with increased risk (pre-diabetes)
>or=6.5% Consistent with diabetes

| eAG (mg/dL) | 235 | | (calc) |
| eAG (mmol/L) | 13 | | (calc) |

Fasting

For an accurate measure of your lipid levels, you need to have fasted for around ten to twelve hours before the test. This means no food or liquid except water until you've had your blood drawn. Failing to follow this guideline will give you a false reading and your cholesterol or triglycerides will tend to be higher than if measured after fasting.

Lipid Panel (also known as Lipoprotein Panel)

Lipids are the fats and fatty-substances accumulated in your body.

Cholesterol, Total

This is the calculated total of all the cholesterol in your body. The formula is a little weird, but it goes like this:
   LDL + HDL + (Triglycerides/5) = Total Cholesterol.
   Therefore, the above cholesterol total sum is:
   109 + 36 + (107/5) = 166 (all numbers are rounded up or down).

HDL Cholesterol

HDL stands for High-Density Lipoproteins and they have the highest protein to fat ratio. You might have heard this being called the 'good' cholesterol. The higher the HDL the better. In this test, you can see this person has HDL 'flagged' as low and to the right you see a 'Reference Range' of what the ideal numbers are for this term.

Ideally, HDL will be higher than 60 to be very good, but the starting point for good HDL is making sure it's over 40mg/dL for men and over 50mg/dL for women. Most people I work with generally have low HDL because they've been told to avoid fat for most of their life; in fact, healthy fats increase HDL. So, if your number is low, then it's time to increase the amount of fat you eat.

Lipoproteins are basically special particles of fat surrounded by a single layer of phospholipid molecules. Without getting way too science-y, phospholipid molecules are made up of two fatty acids with a head and a tail, and they basically control what can make up a cell and what doesn't. In this way, they are known to carry LDL cholesterol away from the tissues to the liver to be reused by the body and lower blood cholesterol.

Cholesterol is a waxy substance which is naturally found in the body and mainly produced in the liver. Cholesterol is important to overall good health but as with everything, we need balance.

Triglycerides

Triglycerides are the most common type of fat found in the body. Just as I think LDL has been overrated for its effect on heart disease, triglycerides have been underrated for their effect on heart disease. When I look at a blood test, the first number I tend to look at is the A1c, followed by the triglyceride because this gives me a quick insight into where a person is health-wise.

Triglycerides are what the body uses to transport any extra energy left in your body after the cells have put up that *'closed'* sign to your glucose. If you remember from earlier, the more insulin resistant you become, the more your triglycerides are likely to rise, as well as your fatty deposits in your body, this includes a buildup in the arteries.

High triglycerides are also one of the markers for metabolic syndrome.

LDL Cholesterol

LDL stands for Low-Density Lipoproteins and have been given the moniker 'bad' cholesterol for a very long time - somewhat unfairly in my opinion. LDL is linked to arterial disease because of its potential to cause *inflammation* in the blood vessel walls, and not because LDL clogs them up like poop in a sewer. The trouble with LDL is that it's blamed for things it doesn't do, and it's still one of those medical myths that won't go away, and doctors still freak out over.

Chol/HDLC Ratio

This is the sum for Total Cholesterol divided by your HDL this will give you your ratio score. If you look to the 'Reference Range' to the right, you'll see that the optimal ratio is 5 or lower. Doctors use this as an indicator to see if somebody is potentially more or less at risk of heart disease. The higher the number, the greater the risk.

Non-HDL Cholesterol

This is basically Total Cholesterol minus your HDL cholesterol. To me, this is a better way of looking at your total cholesterol levels rather than the Total Cholesterol including HDL shown above. What makes this a better indicator is because you want to have high HDL cholesterol in your body and if this HDL is lumped in with the overall total, it will make your look cholesterol higher. But higher doesn't necessarily mean bad. However, the Total Cholesterol is usually the main number doctors look at. Which is a mistake in my humble opinion.

Glucose

We've talked a lot about glucose levels in the blood so far, and I hope you now understand what it means. What this glucose test is looking for is what your blood sugar levels are on the day you take it. Below, I'll talk about A1c, but the main difference between the glucose test and the A1c test is that your glucose is measured over one day, and you're A1c is measured over three months.

A healthy zone for glucose levels is between 65-99mg/dL. Once you go over 100mg/dL then there's a very good chance you are insulin resistant. If your glucose is over 100mg.dL, your doctor might run a further blood test to check how high your blood sugar has been over the past three months - this is your A1c test.

The mg/dL after the number are the units and stands for *milligrams per deciliter*.

Hemoglobin A1c

Your Hemoglobin A1c (sometimes known as HgbA1c, HbA1c depending on which lab does your test) shows your average blood sugar levels over the past three months. This number will reflect whether you are diabetic or pre-diabetic.

A1c means Glycated Hemoglobin A (A is for adult). Hemoglobin is a protein found in your blood cells which transports oxygen from your lungs around your body, and it's also coated in glycate (sugar). The percentage number of your A1c is the percentage of your red blood cells that are covered with sugar. Therefore, the higher the percentage, the higher the sugar circulating around your body, and the higher the risk of long-term health problems.

Once a blood cell is glycated (covered in sugar), the cell lives around three to four months, which is why the A1c test shows the average glucose levels over this time. If you're having an A1c test and not a full lipid panel, then you don't need to be fasting.

For people with diabetes, tests are often administered every three, six and twelve-months, and the good thing about these intervals is that it's very possible to reverse your A1c back to normal levels by the next test. This can be a goal to aim for if you're so inclined.

A note of caution if you are African-American or have Mediterranean or Southeast Asian heritage: Around 90% of people have Hemoglobin A, but if there is a history of sickle cell anemia in your family you might have an uncommon form of hemoglobin called a hemoglobin variant. This variant can give you a false positive on your A1c test. I would assume your doctor would be aware of this from your family history and other blood tests you may have had, but if your A1c looks off or doesn't seem to make sense, you might want to talk to your doctor about this.

eAG (mg/dL)

This means your Estimated Average Glucose and is calculated based on your A1c to show your blood glucose levels over the past few months. If you're monitoring your blood at home, you'll be able to see your glucose number in those *milligrams per deciliter*.

For example: your A1c might be 10% on the blood test, but on a monitor, your eAG will show as 240 mg/dL. Basically, the higher the number, the higher the risk.

eAG (mmol/L)

This is pretty much the same as eAG (mg/dL) but the mmol/L means *millimoles per liter* which is a measurement used more in the UK and Europe. Some blood test monitors are made in the EU, thus the mmol/L reading. The easiest way to convert mg/dL to mmol/L is to divide by 18 or to convert mmol/L to mg/dL multiply by 18.

Extras Factors That Are Not in Your Blood Tests

These following measurements won't be shown on your blood test but they're also tests carried out by your doctor and are relevant to your overall health. These two extra tests are also risk factors that establish if you're considered to have metabolic syndrome.

Blood Pressure

You've probably had your blood pressure taken every time you've been to your doctor's office, but the numbers are rarely explained. You might be told it's normal or a little high or low.

So, what's happening? Well, when your blood pressure is taken, you'll get a reading of two numbers, for example, 110/76, or as it's said, 110 over 76. This might also be written down as 110/76 mmHg (mmHg means millimeters (mm) of mercury (Hg) and is a measurement of pressure).

The first number, 110 is the *systolic pressure*, which means the maximum amount of pressure in your arteries when your heart is contracting or squeezing the blood around your body. The second number is *diastolic pressure*, which measures your blood pressure between beats when your heart is resting.

There are six categories of blood pressure you can fall into, but only elevated, hypertension stage 1, hypertension stage 2 and hypertensive crisis are considered risk factors for metabolic syndrome.

Normal

This is where your blood pressure is healthy and around 120/80 or less. You might find your blood pressure is a little lower than this and that will still be considered healthy.

Low

This range *isn't* a risk factor of metabolic syndrome, but it can still be dangerous to you. Low blood pressure will be below 90/60. Often people have low blood pressure when they are dehydrated.

Elevated

In this range you'll be around 120-129 systolic, and 80 or less diastolic. At this point, you are beginning to be at risk of high blood pressure.

Hypertension Stage 1

This is when your blood pressure is consistently around 130-139 systolic, and 80-89 diastolic. At this stage your doctor will most likely talk to you about lifestyle changes (weight loss, exercise) and possibly prescribe blood pressure medication.

Hypertension Stage 2

This is when your blood pressure is consistently 140/90 or higher. At this stage, your doctor is very likely to prescribe a combination of blood pressure medications as well as encouraging lifestyle changes.

Hypertensive Crisis

This is where you will probably require medical attention. When your blood pressure is 180/120 or higher you could start experiencing some signs of organ damage such as chest pains, backache, shortness of breath and blurred vision.

Your blood pressure does change during the day, so depending on when you have a blood pressure test, a few factors can elevate it. Stress is often the first cause for high blood pressure, as many people have what is called 'white coat syndrome'. This is when faced with a doctor or clinician, anxiety drives blood pressure up. You might not even realize this is happening but is very common.

Rushing to an appointment, fighting traffic, climbing stairs before the test, or having a particularly stressful, or busy day can also lead to higher than normal readings. My tip - if you're going to have your blood pressure taken and you know your heart is beating a little fast from rushing or anxiety, just ask for a moment, close your eyes and breath slowly and deeply for a minute.

Alternatively, ask your doctor to take or retake your blood pressure at the end of your meeting, because many times people are more anxious in the beginning but after talking with the doctor they start to relax, so your blood pressure will likely be lower at the end of the meeting than at the start.

Waist Circumference

This is a straightforward process, but not one that is routinely done by doctors in the US (which is odd as this is one of the first risk factors of metabolic syndrome, but I digress). When your waist circumference is taken, what your doctor is looking for is *abdominal obesity*, also known as *central obesity*. This is when there's clearly a build-up of fat around the abdominal area to the extent that it can be having negative effects on your health. Abdominal obesity is measured at 40 inches and above in men, and greater than 35 inches for women.

This excess abdominal fat is also associated with high levels of triglycerides, LDL cholesterol, and low HDL cholesterol. Often the excess body fat around the belly will feel hard to the touch and can be a major contributor to problems such as heart attacks, strokes, high blood pressure, and diabetes.

The only issue I have with measuring the waist circumference is that somebody who's 6 feet 4" is likely to have a larger waist than somebody who's 5 feet 6". So, in some ways, even though a higher waistline measurement is classed as a risk factor for metabolic syndrome, if you're a big person, this one might go against you. You may not be excessively fat, just built with a lot of abdominal muscle.

Hopefully, this helps you understand what all the terms in your lab work mean because it is easy to feel a little lost in the whole medical processes. To further your understanding, let's look at a few examples of what all this looks like in practice, and at the end, I hope you'll be an expert in reading your own blood work.

Blood Test Examples

Below are seven different example of lipid panels. Feel free to jump to the blood test which best describes your situation.

1. Blood work shows they are diabetic with no other risk factors.
2. Blood work shows they are diabetic with additional risk factors.
3. Blood work shows they are prediabetic with no other risk factors.
4. Blood work shows they are prediabetic with additional risk factors.
5. Blood work shows the minimum three risk factors for metabolic syndrome.
6. Blood work shows all five risk factors for metabolic syndrome.
7. Blood work is healthy.

I've also labeled these as male or female results, just because there's a difference between metabolic syndrome HDL risk factors between the sexes, but the rest of the rangers are going to be similar.

1. Diabetic Without Other Risk Factors (Female Results)

Lipid Panel	Result	Flag	Reference Range
CHOLESTEROL, TOTAL	221	?HIGH	125-200 mg/dL
HDL CHOLESTEROL	(63)		> OR = 46 mg/dL
TRIGLYCERIDES	148		< 150 mg/dL
LDL-CHOLESTEROL	128		< 130 mg/dL (calc)
CHOL/HDLC RATIO	3.5		< OR = 5.0 mg/dL (calc)
NON HDL CHOLESTEROL	158		mg/dL (calc)

Target for non-HDL cholesterol is 30 mg/dL higher than LDL cholesterol target.

Hemoglobin A1c with eAG

HEMOGLOBIN A1C	10.1	HIGH	<5.7% of total Hgb

For the purpose of screening for the presence of diabetes
<5.7% Consistent with the absence of diabetes
5.7-6.4% Consistent with increased risk (pre-diabetes)
>or=6.5% Consistent with diabetes

eAG (mg/dL)	243	(calc)
eAG (mmol/L)	13.5	(calc)

Extras Not Shown

- Blood Pressure: 110/75 (in a normal healthy range).
- Waist Measurement: 39" (just inside a healthy range for a woman).

Summary

In all the blood tests you'll see a column called 'FLAG'. This is where you will be notified whether something is LOW, HIGH, or left blank for the normal healthy range. For this blood test, we can see two things that jump out from the 'FLAG' column as HIGH but only one of those is really a problem which is why it's important that you learn to read your own labs.

Unfortunately, there's little nuance or context in blood tests. The computer reads the numbers and spits out the outcome, regardless of what it means. If you notice I've circled the HDL number, which is 63 and makes that HDL number very, very good because for women a level of over 50mg/dL is considered good.

However, when this test calculates the total cholesterol as 221, that total is flagged as high, when it's high only because the HDL is good. This is why I said I prefer non-HDL cholesterol indicator as the better number for reading total cholesterol because it takes into consideration that some people do have high HDL.

When it comes to this blood test, you can completely ignore that first flag because without this HDL being nice and high, this person wouldn't have been flagged. Plus, we can see all her cholesterol and triglyceride numbers are healthy.

The second flag, unfortunately, *does* highlight a significant problem. This person has an A1c of 10.1% and that's high (I've seen much, much higher).

The interesting thing about this blood test (and it is quite an unusual blood test just due to her lipids looking fine), is that I suspect she is probably an athlete or a vegetarian/vegan of some kind. The reason for this, as I've mentioned before, is that you don't need to be overweight or have bad cholesterol to be diabetic. What this blood test tells me is this person is generally healthy. However, she consumes far too many carbohydrates, which typically happens with vegetarians or vegans as they eat a lot of fruit, bread, legumes, and rice. Or they could be an athlete who eats a lot of carbohydrates from rice, pasta, energy drinks and bars to give them energy to work out.

Most of the time you won't see a blood test like this. Typically, if you have a high A1c which puts you in the diabetic range, there's usually other risk factors associated with the blood test.

2. Diabetic with Other Risk Factors (Male Results)

Lipid Panel	Result	Flag	Reference Range
CHOLESTEROL, TOTAL	302	HIGH	125-200 mg/dL
HDL CHOLESTEROL	28	LOW	> OR = 46 mg/dL
TRIGLYCERIDES	250	HIGH	< 150 mg/dL
LDL-CHOLESTEROL	224	HIGH	< 130 mg/dL (calc)
CHOL/HDLC RATIO	10.7		< OR = 5.0 mg/dL (calc)
NON HDL CHOLESTEROL	274		mg/dL (calc)

Target for non-HDL cholesterol is 30 mg/dL higher than LDL cholesterol target.

Hemoglobin A1c with eAG

HEMOGLOBIN A1C	9.8	HIGH	<5.7% of total Hgb

For the purpose of screening for the presence of diabetes
<5.7% Consistent with the absence of diabetes
5.7-6.4% Consistent with increased risk (pre-diabetes)
>or=6.5% Consistent with diabetes

eAG (mg/dL)	235	(calc)
eAG (mmol/L)	13	(calc)

Extras Not Shown

- Blood Pressure: 155/97 (Hypertension Stage 2).
- Waist Measurement: 56" (unhealthy range for a man).

Summary

It's clear this person's blood and overall health is in a bad way. I suspect this man will have been prescribed multiple medications for blood pressure, cholesterol, and diabetes.

We can see everything in his test is outside of healthy ranges. Having low HDL on top of everything else really does put this person at risk of heart disease or stroke. To me, I would expect a big lifestyle change to be the only thing that would reverse this blood work.

My guess is this man is almost guaranteed to have *Obstructive Sleep Apnea* (OSA), and this could be one of the primary reasons for the high numbers. The reason I say this is when we don't sleep well or have interrupted sleep, every facet of our health is impacted (OSA was covered in the Five Pillars of Good Health).

As bad as this looks, most of these numbers can be back in a healthy range in about six months. Six months of consistency and care for oneself rather than a lifetime on medication and poor health, which is a pretty good deal, I think.

3. Prediabetic Without Other Risk Factors (Female Results)

Lipid Panel	Result	Flag	Reference Range
CHOLESTEROL, TOTAL	166		125-200 mg/dL
HDL CHOLESTEROL	50		> OR = 46 mg/dL
TRIGLYCERIDES	79		< 150 mg/dL
LDL-CHOLESTEROL	100		< 130 mg/dL (calc)
CHOL/HDLC RATIO	3.3		< OR = 5.0 mg/dL (calc)
NON HDL CHOLESTEROL	116		mg/dL (calc)

Target for non-HDL cholesterol is 30 mg/dL higher than LDL cholesterol target.

Hemoglobin A1c with eAG

HEMOGLOBIN A1C	5.8	HIGH	<5.7% of total Hgb

For the purpose of screening for the presence of diabetes
<5.7% Consistent with the absence of diabetes
5.7-6.4% Consistent with increased risk (pre-diabetes)
>or=6.5% Consistent with diabetes

eAG (mg/dL)	120	(calc)
eAG (mmol/L)	66	(calc)

Extras Not Shown

- Blood Pressure: 120/79 (in a normal healthy range).
- Waist Measurement: 34" (in a healthy range).

Summary

In this example, we can see the 'High' flag showing this person has just tipped into the pre-diabetic range. With a blood glucose level of 5.8%, this number is just above the healthy reference range of <5.7%, which is the threshold for healthy blood.

When I look at this blood work, I'm really encouraged that this person will be able to reverse that 5.8% very quickly because the rest of her blood test is really very good.

We can also see her blood pressure and waist circumference are also within a healthy range, so although she has been diagnosed with prediabetes, she's in decent shape and could probably reverse that A1c within a month.

4. Prediabetic with Other Risk Factors (Female Results)

Lipid Panel	Result	Flag	Reference Range
CHOLESTEROL, TOTAL	264	HIGH	125-200 mg/dL
HDL CHOLESTEROL	32	LOW	> OR = 46 mg/dL
TRIGLYCERIDES	160	HIGH	< 150 mg/dL
LDL-CHOLESTEROL	200	HIGH	< 130 mg/dL (calc)
CHOL/HDLC RATIO	8.3		< OR = 5.0 mg/dL (calc)
NON HDL CHOLESTEROL	232		mg/dL (calc)

Target for non-HDL cholesterol is 30 mg/dL higher than LDL cholesterol target.

Hemoglobin A1c with eAG

HEMOGLOBIN A1C	6.2	HIGH	<5.7% of total Hgb

For the purpose of screening for the presence of diabetes
<5.7% Consistent with the absence of diabetes
5.7-6.4% Consistent with increased risk (pre-diabetes)
>or=6.5% Consistent with diabetes

eAG (mg/dL)	148	(calc)
eAG (mmol/L)	8.2	(calc)

Extras Not Shown

- Blood Pressure: 132/82 (this shows Hypertension Stage 1).

- Waist Measurement: 43" (unhealthy range).

Summary

If you compare this pre-diabetic result with the previous one, you'll see some very disturbing differences. As well as having a higher A1c of 6.2% this person also has seven other risk factors which can lead to significant health problems.

These risk factors are:
- High total cholesterol
- High LDL cholesterol
- Low HDL cholesterol
- High triglycerides
- High A1c
- High blood pressure
- High waist measurement

When somebody receives a document like this with the word HIGH in red all over the place it can be very concerning. When I look at this, I can see this person does have some work to do but it really isn't going to take long to get everything back into healthy ranges, and here's why.

The two main things I'm concerned about are the high A1c and the high triglycerides. The LDL cholesterol I don't care so much about as it's not off-the-charts high. Essentially, we have two main things to adjust, and if we take care of those two things the rest of the HIGH flagged risk factors will also reduce as a by-product.

The way we changed her blood panel was to quickly reduce her sugar and carbohydrates, and this was as simple as not drinking soda and fruit juice throughout the day. I then recommend a well-balanced diet of moderate protein and fats as the priority because doing this means she lost weight steadily over several months.

By losing around fifteen to twenty pounds, the waist circumference came down to below 40" and by losing that fat from her middle, her triglycerides, which are what create that fat, were released from the body, therefore her triglycerides went down. This extra loss of body fat and sugar from her blood reduced her blood sugar and LDL cholesterol.

Finally, by eating a diet of good healthy fats, her HDL went up into a healthy range. A few sensible changes make all the difference.

For most people, this change can take as little as a few months, and the outcome is healthy clean blood. It really is that simple.

5. Three Risk Factor Metabolic Syndrome (Male Results)

Lipid Panel	Result	Flag	Reference Range
CHOLESTEROL, TOTAL	280	HIGH	125-200 mg/dL
HDL CHOLESTEROL	36	LOW	> OR = 46 mg/dL
TRIGLYCERIDES	287	HIGH	< 150 mg/dL
LDL-CHOLESTEROL	187	HIGH	< 130 mg/dL (calc)
CHOL/HDLC RATIO	7.7		< OR = 5.0 mg/dL (calc)
NON HDL CHOLESTEROL	244		mg/dL (calc)

Target for non-HDL cholesterol is 30 mg/dL higher than LDL cholesterol target.

| GLUCOSE | 106 | HIGH | 65 - 99 mg/dL |

Extras Not Shown

- Blood Pressure: 98/79 (in a normal healthy range).
- Waist Measurement: 37" (in a healthy range).

Summary

As you can see, the metabolic syndrome blood test is a little different, as A1c isn't tested for. Instead, there is a glucose test.

The interesting thing about this test is that even though there are five flags in the blood test results, when it comes to our metabolic syndrome blood tests, we're only looking at three things: high glucose, low HDL, and high triglycerides, as these are three of the risk factors for metabolic syndrome. The other two risk factors come in the form of waist measurement and blood pressure in the Extra section.

The other high results in the blood test are worth taking note of but for our purposes of lifestyle change, I'm not concerned about those numbers. Remember, LDL is not a main concern, it just isn't as important as the others - even if you've been told otherwise.

Clearly high blood sugar is starting to take its toll on this person's body, and he is clearly insulin resistant. His triglycerides are extremely high, and this tells me his body is starting to struggle with removing the amount of glucose in the blood, and it won't be long before he starts seeing more issues with his blood.

One thing I do have in the back of my mind is that this man may have hereditary high cholesterol and triglycerides running in his family because the waist measurement isn't as excessively high as I'd expect with triglycerides that elevated. Even if that's the case, he still needs to take care of reducing carbs and increasing healthy fats to start reversing his condition.

With his glucose levels at 106, this again is a marker that his blood is starting to struggle and if he was to take the blood test again in three months, there's a good chance that if doesn't make any changes he'll be diagnosed at the very least with prediabetes.

6. All Five Risk Factor Metabolic Syndrome (Male Results)

Lipid Panel	Result	Flag	Reference Range
CHOLESTEROL, TOTAL	165		125-200 mg/dL
HDL CHOLESTEROL	31	LOW	> OR = 46 mg/dL
TRIGLYCERIDES	180	HIGH	< 150 mg/dL
LDL-CHOLESTEROL	98		< 130 mg/dL (calc)
CHOL/HDLC RATIO	5.3		< OR = 5.0 mg/dL (calc)
NON HDL CHOLESTEROL	134		mg/dL (calc)

Target for non-HDL cholesterol is 30 mg/dL higher than LDL cholesterol target.

| GLUCOSE | 103 | HIGH | 65 - 99 mg/dL |

Extras Not Shown

- Blood Pressure: 140/91 (this shows Hypertension Stage 2).
- Waist Measurement: 46" (unhealthy range).

Summary

At first glance, you'd be forgiven for thinking that it looks better than the previous one of three factors of metabolic syndrome but this one is actually a lot worse. Another reason why taking blood tests at face value isn't always a good idea.

Here we see his glucose levels are just above healthy, which is not too high and easily rectified. His triglycerides are also not out of control, but what is really worrying is that he has very low HDL, which puts him at a higher risk of heart disease. Couple this to his very high blood pressure then you have somebody who I would be quite concerned for.

These two things alone tell me that this man is probably under a lot of stress much of the time. I would also guess he doesn't eat a lot of food, maybe travels a lot and just grabs a quick snack here and there between traveling and working.

For me, the first thing we'd need to do is put a plan together to get him to eat more and eat more regularly. We'd also have to figure out how to manage his work situation because sometimes that can be the hardest thing to tackle, as he may not be able to change jobs or his workload. But whatever the case, there are plenty of things we can do to get his blood work back on track.

7. Healthy Blood Work (Female Results)

Lipid Panel	Result	Flag	Reference Range
CHOLESTEROL, TOTAL	200		125-200 mg/dL
HDL CHOLESTEROL	52		> OR = 46 mg/dL
TRIGLYCERIDES	136		< 150 mg/dL
LDL-CHOLESTEROL	121		< 130 mg/dL (calc)
CHOL/HDLC RATIO	3.8		< OR = 5.0 mg/dL (calc)
NON HDL CHOLESTEROL	148		mg/dL (calc)

Target for non-HDL cholesterol is 30 mg/dL higher than LDL cholesterol target.

GLUCOSE	90		65 - 99 mg/dL

Extras Not Shown

- Blood Pressure: 118/78 (in a normal healthy range).
- Waist Measurement: 34" (in a healthy range).

Summary

This is what we hope to achieve by cleansing your blood. Everything in normal healthy ranges. Luckily, her HDL wasn't any higher or she would have kicked that unhelpful metric High total cholesterol flag off (silly flag), but overall this is great.

We can see her HDL is over 50 which is good but can always improve. Her triglycerides are low, and her glucose is in the low 90's which I like to see.

Overall, A+.

The Spread of Poor Blood Health

You might have noticed by now that I'm passionate about reversing diabetes, prediabetes and metabolic syndrome. I've seen up-close how it can debilitate and lead to premature death, and I wouldn't wish that on anyone. One of the struggles I have is watching people not take their blood condition seriously, because, let's face it, the government and health care services don't make a big deal of it, so why should we?

But don't be fooled, there is a health crisis in America and the rest of the world and in another 10-15 years, this crisis is going to go off like a bomb unless something is done right now. I'd like to show you why your condition is a big deal and how quickly people are getting sicker.

Let's take diabetes as an example, only because there is a lot more data on this condition. I want to show you some diagrams created by the Centers for Disease Control (CDC) on how quickly the prevalence of diagnosed diabetes has grown amongst adults in the USA from 1995 to 2015 - just twenty years. I'll then show you how much money is spent on researching a *cure* for diabetes, prediabetes, and metabolic syndrome. And finally, I want to show you how much money is made from keeping you sick... sorry, silly mistake. I meant; how much money is made by pharmaceutical companies who are trying to help you cleanse your blood...

Instead of just accepting my opinion about the problem facing you and millions like you, I'm hoping this Government created data is enough to really scare you. My hope is the reality of your condition will be enough to motivate you to make necessary changes in your life to cleanse your blood.

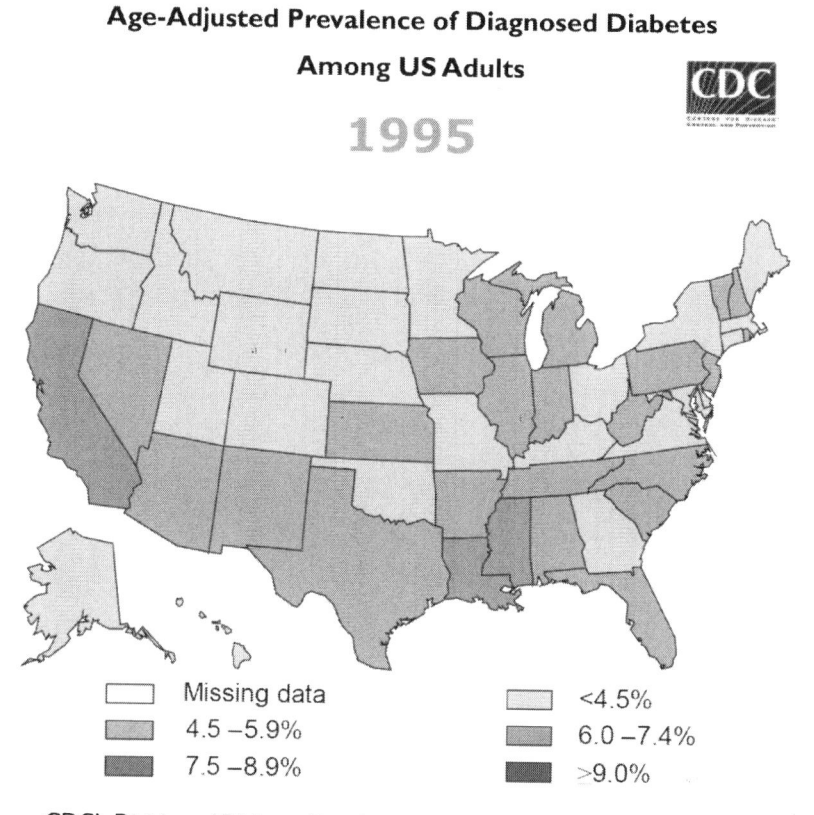

Age-Adjusted Prevalence of Diagnosed Diabetes Among US Adults

1995

☐ Missing data	☐ <4.5%
▨ 4.5–5.9%	▨ 6.0–7.4%
▰ 7.5–8.9%	■ >9.0%

CDC's Division of Diabetes Translation. United States Diabetes Surveillance System available at http://www.cdc.gov/diabetes/data

What we can see from this initial image is that around half the US have at least 4.5% to 7.4% of the adult population diagnosed with diabetes (remember, this is just diagnosed, and we know there are many more who are not diagnosed). At first viewing, this doesn't seem that bad, right? Over half the States have a negligible proportion of the population with diabetes. Clearly, at this point, diabetes isn't out of control, and in theory it would be much easier to create State-wide health strategies to stop the problem getting any worse. Alas, that isn't what happens, which you'll see over the following years.

Age-Adjusted Prevalence of Diagnosed Diabetes Among US Adults
2000

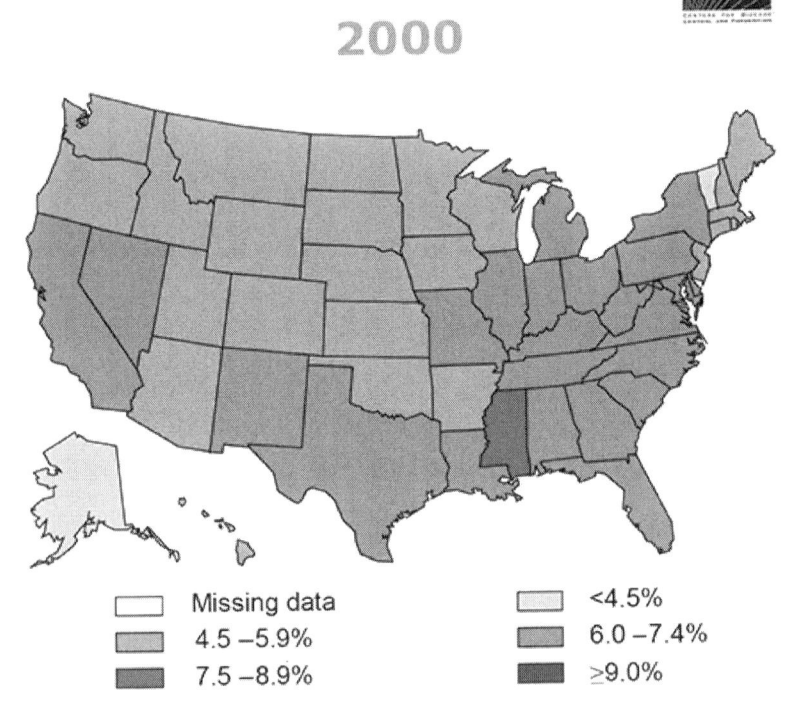

- Missing data
- 4.5 – 5.9%
- 7.5 – 8.9%
- <4.5%
- 6.0 – 7.4%
- ≥9.0%

CDC's Division of Diabetes Translation. United States Diabetes Surveillance System available at http://www.cdc.gov/diabetes/data

In this image, you can see, the reduction in light yellow color throughout the US, except for Vermont and Alaska holding on valiantly against the rising tide of diabetes. Our first darker red State has also appeared in Missouri. This puts the diagnosis in this State for diabetes around 7.5% to 8.9%; that's close to 490,000 people in 2000.

Age-Adjusted Prevalence of Diagnosed Diabetes Among US Adults

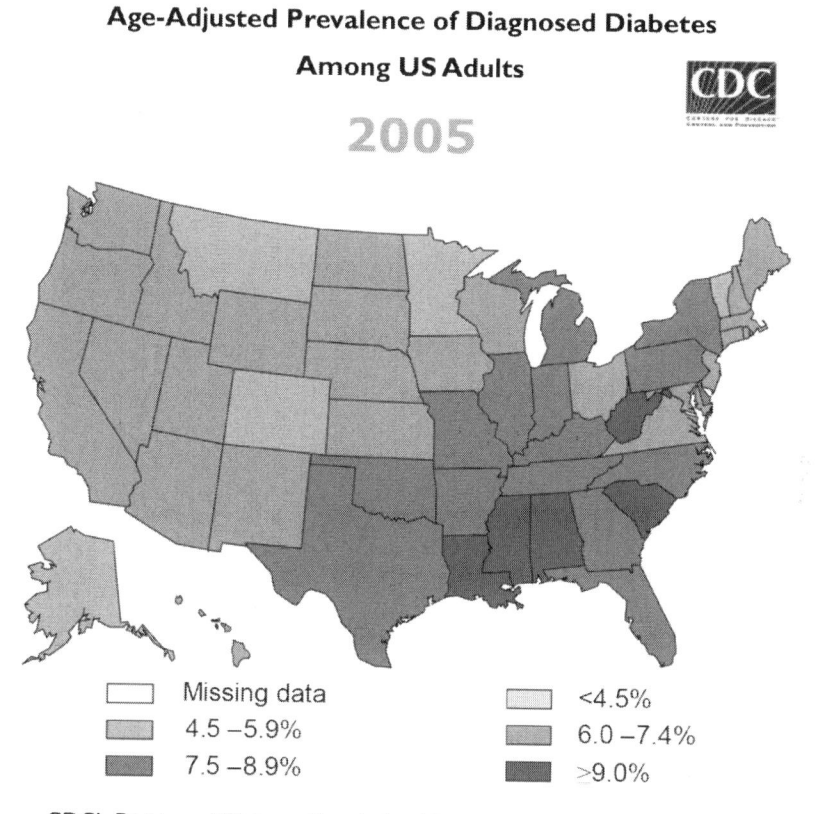

2005

- Missing data
- 4.5 – 5.9%
- 7.5 – 8.9%
- <4.5%
- 6.0 – 7.4%
- ≥9.0%

CDC's Division of Diabetes Translation. United States Diabetes Surveillance System available at http://www.cdc.gov/diabetes/data

Just 5 years after our first red State appears, there seems to be no holding the spread of diabetes back. We also have 5 States with the top percentage of over 9% of the population diagnosed with diabetes. Sadly, they stop recording percentages over 9%. As far as we know in this graphic and over the coming years, the percentage could be and probably is, way higher than 9% of the populations. It wouldn't be a stretch of the imagination to think at least 50% of the population of the red colored States are struggling with diabetes.

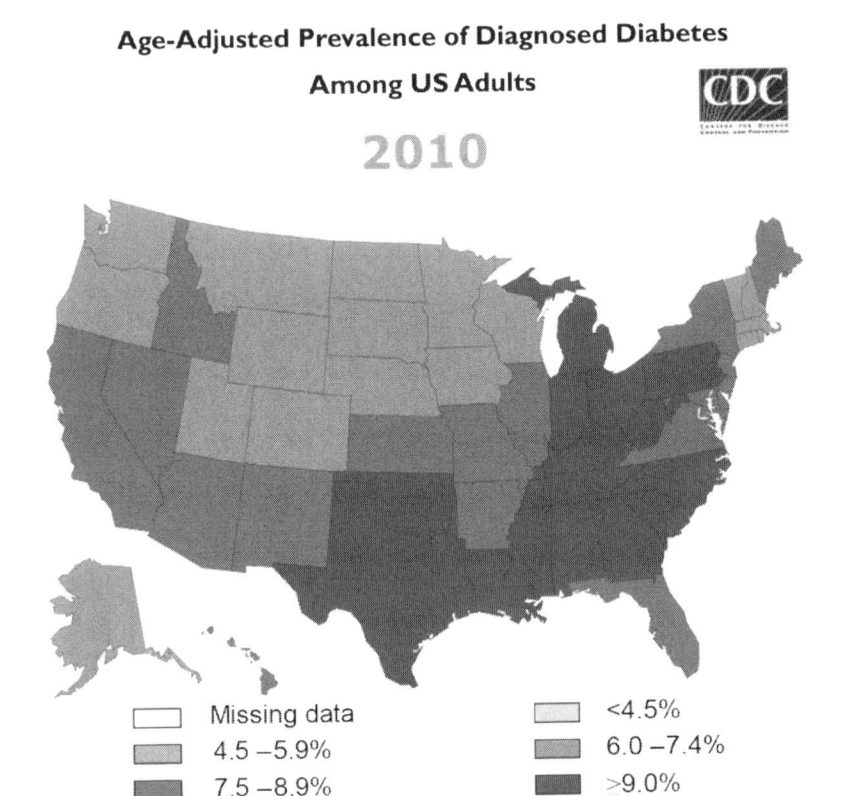

Age-Adjusted Prevalence of Diagnosed Diabetes Among US Adults

2010

- Missing data
- 4.5 – 5.9%
- 7.5 – 8.9%
- <4.5%
- 6.0 – 7.4%
- >9.0%

CDC's Division of Diabetes Translation. United States Diabetes Surveillance System available at http://www.cdc.gov/diabetes/data

In just 5 more years, the amount of high levels of diagnosed diabetes has tripled and no State has less than 6% of their population diagnosed with diabetes.

CLEANSE YOUR BLOOD · 281

Age-Adjusted Prevalence of Diagnosed Diabetes Among US Adults

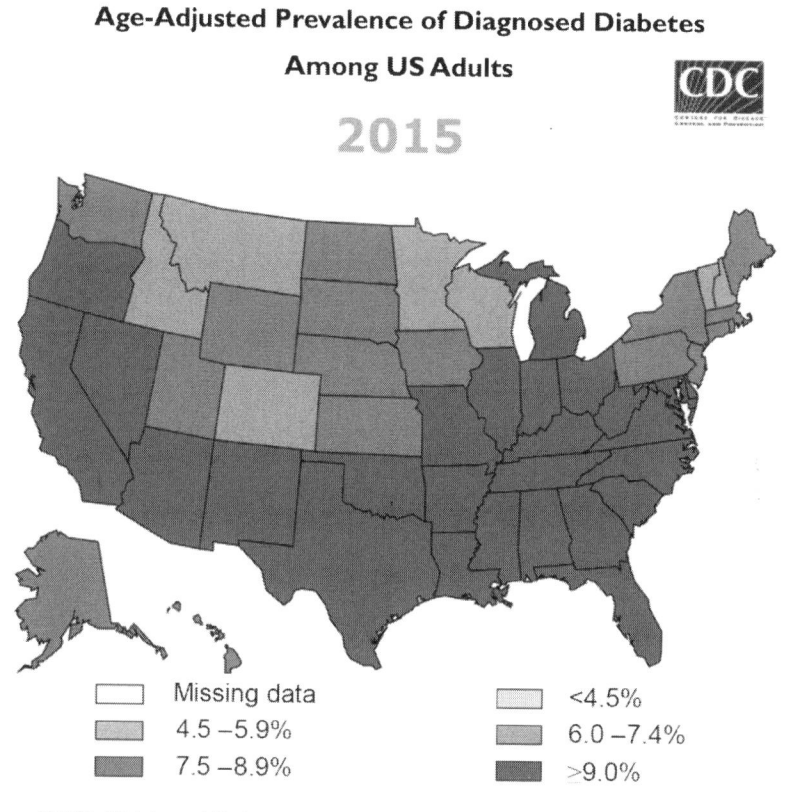

2015

Legend:
- Missing data
- 4.5 – 5.9%
- 7.5 – 8.9%
- <4.5%
- 6.0 – 7.4%
- >9.0%

CDC's Division of Diabetes Translation. United States Diabetes Surveillance System available at http://www.cdc.gov/diabetes/data

The entire US is now experiencing high levels of diagnosed diabetes. In the next 5 years, the entire map will be one solid color if the rise of diabetes isn't addressed in sensible ways.

When I look at these images, not only am I saddened by how quickly the prevalence of diabetes has taken hold, but I also see a population whose health is getting worse because the urgency to correctly address the underlying problems of diabetes is woefully inadequate and outdated. How can so many people be diagnosed with diabetes over such a brief period without any intervention by the government or health care providers? Essentially, these people (and you) have been failed by a failed system.

The Money Machine

Now you've seen the CDC's data on the prevalence of diabetes, let's take a quick look at medication. I mentioned earlier that I don't think medication is a good long-term solution because medication for diabetes, prediabetes and metabolic syndrome do not reverse the condition, they manage and maintain it. If this CDC data showed the rise of cancer and heart disease over the same period of time, there would be a national crisis and a demand for a cure. However, diabetes, prediabetes and metabolic syndrome do not kill people quickly. But and I will show you later in this chapter, these conditions still kill, and I am convinced diabetes, prediabetes and metabolic syndrome are just as much a killer in the USA than cancer and heart disease.

You see, the problem with your condition is that it can be managed and maintained in its current state for years. And if something can be managed, that means medication is involved.

If we take insulin as an example, the price of it has nearly tripled in the past ten years. In 2002 the cost was $4.34 per milliliter of insulin. And in 2012 the cost was $12.92.[29] So, what does this tell us? It tells us the demand for insulin is so high that manufacturers can keep raising the price because they know people have to use their product.

For some people, injecting insulin does indeed save their life and is important to take it, but why recommend a drug that continues to maintain a problem and doesn't fix it?

Another popular drug for managing and maintaining these conditions is called Metformin. This is typically the first-line oral glucose-lowering drug many people are given to manage early-stage diabetes, prediabetes, and metabolic syndrome.

In the USA Metformin is currently the fifth most commonly-prescribed drug, and it's the number one drug dispensed in the diabetes market. In 2008 51.6 million prescriptions were written for the drug, which increased to 61.6 million in 2012.[30] At a monthly cost per prescription of between $4 - $10, we're talking big money for the pharmaceutical industry again. My guess is new research will show these prescriptions are now around the 80 million mark. That's a lot of medication and a lot of money being spent on a condition which can be reversed in as little as three months.

List of the Top Ten US Killers in 2016

Your condition also doesn't garner the same kind of research dollars as many other diseases or conditions. Don't get me wrong, other issues like cancer and heart disease are both horrible, and I wouldn't wish that on anyone but with so many people in the US with your blood condition and the epidemic spreading quickly, you'd think there would be a lot of money spent on finding a significant cure.

Well, let's look at the research dollars spent on the top ten killers in the US in 2016 to get an idea of what's deemed more deserving of research.

- Heart disease
- Cancer
- Chronic Lower Respiratory Disease
- Accidents
- Stroke or Cerebrovascular Disease
- Alzheimer's
- Diabetes
- Influenza and Pneumonia
- Kidney Disease
- Suicide

Overall, this is a bad list and I know what you're thinking, accidents at number 4; I know, that's quite the surprise. Also, prediabetes and metabolic syndrome are nowhere to be seen on this list because people don't usually die from those conditions... or do they?

Let's look a little closer to see if we can discover something about what's behind many of these bigger, killer diseases.

1. Heart Disease & Coronary Heart Disease (CHD)

- Total deaths from heart disease and CHD per year: 614,348
- Total deaths from CHD alone: 370,000
- Money spent on research: $1.7 billion[^^]

There are several reasons why people have heart disease but the main reason for Coronary Heart Disease is caused by plaque buildup on the artery walls. This narrows the artery and stops blood from flowing freely to the heart. This process is called atherosclerosis and 370,000 people die from it each year.

What's interesting about CHD is that it's one of the risk factors for metabolic syndrome, is low HDL which can lead to a build-up of plaque and inflammation in the artery walls. That's right, if you have metabolic syndrome then you are more likely to die from CHD. Without realizing it. If you have metabolic syndrome and it's left unchecked, you are far more at risk than you might have known.

2. Cancer

- Total Deaths per year: 591,700
- Estimated people living with cancer: 14.7 million
- Money spent on research: $5.389 billion[^^]

Cancer is one of those diseases most of us are afraid of. The idea of being told by a doctor that you have cancer is a terrible thought. Lung cancer accounts for the most cancer deaths in both men and women, and a substantial cause of that cancer is cigarette smoking (yeah, that thing that is just taxed instead of banned).

However, the World Cancer Research Fund (WCRF) estimate around *one-third* of cancer cases in the US is related to being overweight, obese and having poor nutrition. Aha! If this is the case, then potentially one-third of cancers can be avoided, because being overweight and obese is another risk factor of metabolic syndrome and can be reversed. That's potentially 197,233 deaths that could be avoided by a few simple lifestyle changes. Very sad.

One other thing: look at how much money is spent on research for cancer. The number one killer in the US is heart disease, but the research for that is $1.7 billion compared to $5.4 billion for cancer. These dollar amounts are kind of indicate of how 'sexy' a type of disease is to big pharma.

3. Chronic Lower Respiratory Disease (CLRD) or Lung Disease

- Total deaths per Year: 147,101
- Estimated people diagnosed with a form of CLRD: 12.7 million
- Money spent on research: $1.6 billion^^

Chronic Lower Reparatory Disease is a collection of lung diseases which cause breathing-related issues, the primary one being Chronic Obstructive Pulmonary Disease (COPD). About 80% of all CLRD can be attributed to smoking (again with the smoking!).

4. Accidents

- Total deaths per year: 135,928

What can I say... just be careful out there!

5. Stroke or Cerebrovascular Disease

- Total deaths per year: 133,103
- Estimated people who have a stroke in a year: 795,000
- Money spent on research: $828 million^^

Stroke is like Chronic Heart Disease, but instead of blood flow being slowed to the heart, this time the blood flow is slowed to the brain. Just like Chronic Heart Disease, this is another disease that can easily be linked to metabolic syndrome, as most strokes are due to high blood pressure and unhealthy lifestyle choices leading to being overweight and having high cholesterol.

Most strokes afflict people 65 years and older, but you do become more at risk from the age of 45 years onwards.

6. Alzheimer's

- Total deaths per year: 93,541
- Estimated people living with Alzheimer's: 5.5 million
- Money spent on research: $2.09 billion (Inc. Alzheimer's-related dementia) ^^

Alzheimer's is one type of dementia but similar in the symptoms to dementia. For people with Alzheimer's, damage to the neurons in the brain eventually impairs the person's ability to do many of the basic daily functions we take for granted like swallowing, walking, and remembering. Eventually, as the neurons in the brain die, so will the person.

New research is showing that there is potentially a link between diabetes and Alzheimer's and that Alzheimer's might be part of late-stage diabetes. The theory is that the long-term elevated levels of insulin in the body also affects cognitive brain functioning.

It's early days on this research but there seems to be a clear link emerging between people with diabetes and those who go on to develop Alzheimer's.[31,32,33]

Also, other studies have found a potential link between metabolic syndrome and vascular dementia.[34] I think what we are seeing regarding Alzheimer's is that insulin resistance could be a major contributor to this currently incurable disease.

7. Diabetes

- Deaths caused by diabetes alone: 76,535
- Deaths with diabetes as a contributor: 252,806
- People living with diabetes in the USA: 29.1 million
- People living with prediabetes in the USA: 86 million
- Adults with diagnoses of metabolic syndrome in the USA: 44 million
- Money spent on research: $1.08 billion[^^]

Not only is diabetes itself a killer, but all conditions contribute to heart disease, kidney disease, and stroke. So, including diabetes alone, four of the top ten killers in America are linked to diabetes and metabolic syndrome. That means, diabetes and metabolic syndrome are clearly more than likely connected with these deaths.

One of the most terrifying statistics from the CDC research is that in the year 2013 to 2014 there was a rise of 8.1% cases of death from diabetes alone. Every other top ten disease (except accidents, up 2.8%) went down in that same period. If that's the case, diabetes is the fastest-growing cause of death in the USA, and that is something to be very concerned about.

Another thing to remember is that there are 15.4 million people living with cancer in the US, but 159.1 million living with diabetes, prediabetes and metabolic syndrome. That makes the USA a walking time bomb, and we don't want you to be included in that statistic.

Oh, remember I said to look at the dollar amount spent on research to see which conditions are thought of as sexier and more important? Well, diabetes receives just over $1billion for a condition that affects more than 50% of the population of the USA, while cancer receives five times that for something that affects around 5% of the population. I know it's like comparing oranges to apples, and I know cancer can kill people quickly but if nothing is done about the insulin-resistant epidemic in the USA, then all these top ten diseases will be going up exponentially in the next twenty years.

8. Influenza and Pneumonia

- Total deaths per year: 55,227
- Money spent on research: $380 million^^

Influenza is a highly contagious disease usually most prevalent during the winter. Pneumonia can complicate influenza as pneumonia causes inflammation in the lungs. Influenza is often transmitted through coughs and sneezes and leads to fever, headaches, and other symptoms of the flu.

Pneumonia, on the other hand, causes the air sacs in the lungs to fill with liquid and pus, which prevents oxygen from reaching the bloodstream. Without the oxygen, our cells cease to function properly, and death follows.

Very often our lifestyle choices such as poor nutrition and lack of sleep can reduce our immune system and put us more at risk of contracting influenza and pneumonia. All things we can address without medication.

9. Kidney Disease

- Total deaths per year: 48,146
- Money spent on research: $574 million^^

Chronic Kidney Disease (CKD) is most prevalent in people over 70 years old. This condition happens when the kidneys can no longer filter our blood as well as healthy kidneys can, and the waste from this unfiltered blood can lead to several health problems.

One of the problems with CKD is that it's not often detected early because there aren't always clear symptoms but just like many of the diseases here, as well as medication, a change in eating and drinking habits can have a positive effect on the recovery from CKD.

10. Suicide

- Total deaths per year: 42,828
- Money spent on research: $52 million^^

As a therapist, there's a lot I can say about this, but that's for another book.

OK, so you've read about the top American serial killers, but why does this matter? Well, the way I see it, diabetes, prediabetes and metabolic syndrome are not only killers in their own right but I think it's fair to say they have a hand in many other deaths from disease, and that means these conditions really need to be taken way more seriously than they currently are.

The above data is taken from the Centers for Disease Control and Prevention (CDC) research - National Vital Statistics Reports, Vol. 65 No. 4, June 30, 2016

^^ Financial data from U.S. Department of Health & Human Services: Actual funding from grants and contracts across the National Institutes of Health (NIH) for various research, conditions, and disease categories

(RCDC). Published: July 3, 2017. This doesn't include financial data from individual companies conducting research.

PART FIVE:

QUESTIONS

"The art and science of asking questions is the source of all knowledge."
- Thomas Berger

FAQ

Before we come to the end of this book, I want to try and answer questions you still might have. Over the years I've heard many good questions, and below are some of the most common. If there is something I haven't covered or answered in this book regarding your blood condition, I welcome emails. Feel free to contact me and I'll do my best to reply - **cleanseyourblood@drewcoster.com**

These following questions are in no particular order and I hope my answers are useful to you.

"Am I able to have protein shakes for a quick meal or snack?"

Absolutely, yes! I've even added protein powder to the GO proteins. Of course, it would be ideal if you got all your protein needs from whole foods rather than powder and shakes but I would be remiss if I didn't cover the benefits and drawbacks of protein powders and shakes.

I for one often have a protein shake during the day as a meal replacement or snack. I find them to be beneficial to my lifestyle, as well as tasty. But and this is a big but, they can be over-used and relied upon too heavily because they are convenient.

I remember when I first started drinking protein powders back in the 1980's they were bad. They tasted chalky and nasty, mostly because they were made from dried egg. Luckily, these days there's a wide choice of protein powders made from whey, soy, pea, egg (still) and hemp protein.

Research tells us that protein drinks do not satiate us as much as real food, especially at breakfast, and this can also lead to increased appetite through the day.[62] From my experience, I tend to feel hungry about an hour after drinking a shake, so if I have one for a snack it's no problem but if I have one for breakfast I make sure I blend in some avocado and maybe a couple of strawberries to give it added fat and a little more carbs which I feel I need in the morning.

If you think you'd like to try adding protein powder or protein drinks to your plan, I recommend aiming for a good brand like Optimum Nutrition, or My Protein. These have good ratios of protein to carbs and ideally, you'll be looking at protein labels to get a good idea of what you are drinking. Most good protein powders will have 22g or more of protein with 4-7g of carbs or less. If a protein powder has less protein and more carbs, I don't recommend it. Many bigger known store brands are not as good, so do check that label.

"I'm a vegetarian and I find getting enough protein in my diet hard, is there anything more I can do?"

I've got to be honest, being a vegetarian is going make eating enough protein a challenge unless you use a protein powder supplement. The one I recommend is Vega Protein as they are good quality products, but you can also find alternative proteins in Trader Joe's. Just make sure the protein doesn't contain a lot of carbs.

You can also have any seafood, especially salmon, which is great. Hemp seeds, pumpkin or other seeds are good and can be eaten on their own or added to other foods. Tofu, tempeh, or veggie burgers make a nice change (Morning Star Farms have some great veggie burgers). Edamame or chickpeas are also good, but all peas and beans contain a lot of carbs, so even though they might be a staple, portion control still needs to be moderate - but they will offer more protein.

If you eat eggs and dairy, then eat as many eggs as you can, and whole or 2% plain Greek yogurt or cottage cheese are also excellent protein options.

"Doesn't Eating Fat Make Me Fat?"

The idea that fat, especially saturated fat, was bad for your heart came from a study led by Ancel Keys back in the 1950's. The trouble is this research was quite flawed. He had his own agenda which he wanted his research to prove, and that is never a good start for research. His premise was to show how countries whose populations ate a lot of fat had increased cholesterol, which he claimed led to higher rates of coronary heart disease. It's an interesting story which you might want to look-up, but I'll keep it short. Unfortunately, he didn't use all the data he collected, only that which fit his theory. And in doing so he helped shape the view on fat and cholesterol as being bad for the next 50 years. Thus, sending us on the obesity and diabetic path we are now on. Keys' paper has been fully debunked over the years but it's years too late.

Luckily, we now know this to be wrong but it's an idea which has been in the collective consciousness for so long it has become 'truth', and an accepted 'truth' is hard to shake.

What made this research so ingrained was back in the 1970's is that food manufacturers jumped on this fat-fear and began making food products fat-free which seemed like the answer to our fat-fear prayers.

It was around this time we were also encouraged to eat more grains and pasta because they were supposedly heart healthy but that is far from the actual truth. It's like we all walked into a strange 'mirror universe' where everything became the opposite of what is right and healthy. In this mirror universe, grains are good for you, and fats are bad, so eat more pasta and forget the butter. This is the complete opposite of what we now know to be true.

I don't know about you, but I remembered how the 1990's was like a fat-free zone. There was nothing on the shelves which contained fat. Everything was pasta this, and whole grain that. Even butter was replaced with more synthetic foods claiming to taste 'butter-like' but with less fat (and more chemicals). People wanted butter but were scared to death that one taste would make their hearts explode. And what's happened since then? An obesity and diabetic epidemic that seems to show no signs of slowing down.

As far as I can tell, the more fat removed from food, the more carbohydrates and sugar was added to thicken it and give it taste. The more we ate of that dopamine-creating sugar, the more carbohydrate-sensitive and insulin-resistant people became. There is no other single reason that explains what has happened in the past 50 years to increase obesity and your blood condition than the increase in fat-free foods and the rise of easily available processed products packed with carbs.

"I always thought fruits and vegetables are good for me and I should eat a lot. Are they good for me?"

Well, this statement is both true and false. By now you understand everything you need to know about sugar, carbs, and glucose, so I know you're not surprised to learn that fruits and vegetables *do* offer a lot of health benefits, yet it's important that we get a good balance of these choices. As the WHOA! list tells us, not all fruits and vegetables are created equal for people with diabetes, prediabetes, and metabolic syndrome. Essentially fruit and vegetables are made up of fiber and fructose, and fructose is a fruit sugar. Fiber is great for us and has many health benefits such as providing good colon health, and fiber also helps to push fat out of our body, but the downside of fruit is the fructose.

As I mentioned many times, all carbohydrates are broken down into glucose in the blood. Fructose is a simple sugar, the same as glucose and sucralose - basically, if it has '*ose*' at the end, you know it's a sugar. The main concern with having too much fructose is that unlike glucose, where virtually every cell in the body can use it, only the liver can break down fructose in any significant way. What happens to fructose in the liver is complicated but the two main things we're concerned about from the breakdown of fructose are triglycerides and uric acid.

Uric acid is usually broken down by the kidneys and expelled through urine. However, like so many things in this book, there's always another dimension to these bodily functions. If the body produces more uric acid than the kidneys can cope with, then solid crystals can form within joints, leading to things like gout, kidney stones, and kidney failure.

So, are fruits and vegetables good for you? Sure, but like most things, in moderation - and by moderation, I'm talking about one piece of fruit a day.

In the 1800's and early 1900's fruit and fructose were scarce, with the average American eating around 15g of fructose a day from fruit and vegetables. That's the equivalent of an apple and some veg like a cup of cabbage. Today it's estimated that the average American eats around 55g of fructose, with adolescents eating around 75g. Personally, I think this is a low estimation; and I'd guess it's easily north of 100g of fructose a day if we realistically look at the amount of fruit, or fructose-based foods (bread, juice, frozen meals, candy, flavored yogurts, soda) many people eat today.

"I really don't like vegetables. Is there something else I can eat to get enough fiber, while still low in carbohydrates?"

Firstly, if you were sitting in front of me in my office, I might tell you to grow up and just eat your vegetables as there really isn't any reason to not eat them. I know you may not have eaten them throughout your life, but before you try anything else, give them another try. A lot of people don't like vegetables because they have too much of a sweet tooth, so vegetables just taste bland. However, as you reduce your carbohydrates and sugar intake, your taste buds will change, and you'll be able to taste vegetables much more.

Whatever your reason for not liking veg, you need to experiment and just eat some. It's not that you have to like them all, just choose a few that you can experiment with. You might start with some of my favorites - cauliflower, green beans, mushrooms, and peppers - as these vegetables don't have a strong flavor and are easy to roast in the oven.

I grew up with my mother boiling every vegetable in sight and I despised them until I was in my twenties, when I discovered how to cook vegetables the way I like them. I've enjoyed them ever since. I still have certain vegetables that I don't like, and I avoid those, but I'm also surprised at how many different varieties of vegetables I try and discover I enjoy. You might also like your vegetables raw and crunchy instead of cooked. Try broccoli, jicama, and celery raw with some salt or a dip, like hummus or cream cheese.

The other tip I can give you is to put a Double Cupped Palm portion of leafy greens on your plate, then add your hot food on top. This might be a steak with a few sweet potatoes on the greens. This allows the leafy greens to absorb some of the meat juice and gives them a little extra flavor. By doing this, you're adding leafy greens for added fiber, but they're not the main focus of your meal as they would be if you had a salad. And as you eat the steak, you won't really notice the greens.

As for alternative fiber sources, you can always have some blackberries or raspberries, as they are typically low in sugar and high in fiber. Avocado and edamame are also a good source of fiber. You could also add a tablespoon of flaxseed meal or chia seeds to a plain Greek yogurt for added fiber. As a last resort, there are fiber supplements you can take, although I'm not a fan of these as it's way too easy to take too many. These supplements can lead to constipation, which is the opposite of what fiber should really do for you. If you do think supplementation is right for you, I suggest talking with your doctor.

"There seems to be a lot of eggs in this plan, and I thought eggs were bad for you. What's the truth?"

I hope by now you've realized that fats are good, and carbs are not so good for your blood. The whole egg debate was centered around the fear of cholesterol leading to heart disease, but as we now know, cholesterol in food doesn't lead to heart disease.[39,40] Eggs really are a nutritional powerhouse, not only because they contain healthy fat and protein, but they also contain eye-protecting nutrients like lutein and zeaxanthin, which is eggcellent news (it had to be done…). These two nutrients have been linked to a better reduction of photo-oxidative stress and macular degeneration in the retina, which is especially important as we get older.[78,79] So, eggs are good in every way possible and I encourage you to enjoy them whenever you like.

"French fries are made from potato, so why are they included in the NO section?"

Ah, French fries... I too love fries, and I remember the first time I had real fries in the South of France when I was 10 years old. They were the most amazing tasting fries I think I'd ever had up to that point, so I totally understand any frustration with fries being in the NO section.

The problem with fries isn't so much that they're made from potato. It's because fries are, well, fried, which makes them ultimately unhealthy. Most fried foods are cooked in vegetable oil which can be high in trans fats, you know how I feel about trans fats.

The other problem with fries is that restaurants like McDonald's briefly dip their fries in a sugar solution which gives them their color, and Burger King dip theirs in a starchy batter before frying to give them a crunch. As you can probably tell, these two additions to fries increase unnecessary carbs.

I don't know if you've ever looked at the ingredients in a McDonalds or Burger King French fry but if you do, you'll realize you're not just eating potato.

McDonalds French Fries Ingredients
Potatoes, Vegetable Oil (Canola Oil, Corn Oil, Soybean Oil, Hydrogenated Soybean Oil, Natural Beef Flavor [Wheat and Milk Derivatives]*), Dextrose, Sodium Acid Pyrophosphate (Maintain Color), Salt.
*Natural beef flavor contains hydrolyzed wheat and hydrolyzed milk as starting ingredients.

Burger King French Fries Ingredients
Potatoes, Soybean Oil or Canola and Palm Oil, Modified Potato Starch, Rice Flour, Potato Dextrin, Salt, Leavening (Disodium Dihydrogen Pyrophosphate, Sodium Bicarbonate), Dextrose, Xanthan Gum, Sodium Acid Pyrophosphate added to preserve natural color.

Looking at these two lists of ingredients you'd be forgiven for feeling betrayed by so much rubbish being added to a simple potato. You not only get the potato, but you get a whole lot of unhealthy GMO oils and a lot of added sugar, wheat, and even rice flour.

And lastly, there's the portion size of fries. Even in a medium portion, there are around 12 sugar cubes worth of blood-busting carbs. This is why I say you could have a few for taste but not more than that. By all means, make your own oven-baked fries from only potato or sweet potato because you can still have a good portion. Just avoid fries that are fried.

"I love chocolate and can't see myself giving it up. Is there an alternative I can have?"

I understand how you feel, and what I do is choose a bar of good chocolate, usually around 70% cocoa. I'll sometimes get a bar of Green & Blacks Organic Dark Chocolate (sometimes the mint) and have a square or two in the evening after dinner if I feel the need for something dessert-like. By having a higher cocoa percentage, you're more likely getting a quality chocolate that isn't packed full of sugar and milk. 70% dark chocolate also tends to be a little bitter which makes it harder to overeat. Just remember, if chocolate is your trigger food and you can't stick to one or two pieces maximum, you need to remove that chocolate from your house.

"I really can't drink 100oz of water a day, I just feel so bloated from it. Am I okay drinking less?"

Sure. My ideal is around 100oz, but even if you get around 60-80oz then you'll be doing great. Just make sure you do drink water or herbal tea throughout the day, and remember, caffeine drinks like tea and coffee don't count towards your total. If you are drinking a lot of caffeinated tea and not much water, then focus on switching this around. Getting 100oz isn't essential but it is a respectable number to aim for. Check out the tips for drinking more water in the Five Pillars section if you still need a little boost.

"I'm in a wheelchair and find it hard to do high intensity exercise. Any suggestions?"

Swimming is always a great form of exercise to raise your heart rate. There are also many wheelchair users who do CrossFit and I'm sure if you contact your local CrossFit gym, they will be more than happy to help you. The fitness equipment manufacturer Concept2 can also modify rowing machines to be used with your chair. They can be contacted at info@concept2.com.

"I'm worried about how I'm going to eat on vacation. Do you have any tips?"

Hopefully, you take vacations and enjoy them. If you do, then they can be a real challenge because if you're like me, then I tend to have an *it's a vacation so I can just enjoy myself* type of attitude. Consequently, what happens is I eat a little more junk food than I typically would. I know this isn't ideal but I'm enjoying myself on vacation and food is an important part of that equation. Do I sometimes overdo it? Yes. Do I know I'm doing it? Yes. Do I continue when I get home or after the vacation is over? No. I like to be honest with myself and at times I struggle with vacations and that's okay. I'm aware of it and over time I find a happy medium that works for me. I am a fan of having fun on vacations and I'll tell you why.

Vacations

My advice when it comes to vacations - enjoy yourself. I usually find even if my clients go away and have fun, maybe drink too much and have a few desserts, they come back feeling refreshed and less stressed. This reduction in stress often counteracts the poor food choices. Remember, high blood sugar isn't always about the food you eat but how much you've slept, or how much stress you're under. So, being able to go away, decompress, sleep and rest is going to have a positive effect on lowering your blood sugar and insulin levels naturally. This will help your body find a balance during those times when you do have a little extra fun on vacation.

Public Holidays and Celebrations

Public holidays are a little different from vacations because I find they tend to be more stressful occasions for people because of the social and family aspects. These public holidays are things like Thanksgiving, Halloween, or Christmas. But whatever holiday it is you celebrate, there tends to be a lot more entertaining, a lot of cooking, and a lot of family, and those three things can be a recipe for disaster. I don't know how well you get on with your family but it's not uncommon for people to not look forward to spending time with the in-laws or parents.

My advice for holidays is quite the opposite to vacations. This time I would say be more on your plan than not. This might mean more planning of what you are going to cook if you have a large family gathering. If it's Halloween and you have kids, either buy candy you don't like, or the day after Halloween, take your leftover candy to work and give it to co-workers like a sugar pusher, or simply throw it away. Either way, just get it out of the house. Having candy lying around can be like a red flag to a bull, and you don't want to give yourself any unnecessary temptation.

If you're visiting parents or friends for the holiday, then I advise giving them plenty of warning that there are certain foods you don't eat, and that you'd be happy to bring your own if it's too inconvenient for them to cook something special for you. A lot of my clients think this is being rude but it's not. If you had a peanut allergy that could cause you to go into anaphylactic shock, I'm sure your friends would adjust accordingly, and it's no different with your condition. Eating food, you know isn't good for your blood will do you damage; and that's probably the last thing they, or you, want.

Be clear upfront. Tell them of your nutrition plan, and don't feel embarrassed about it, this is your health after all. I often find people are quite excited about seeing healthy dishes during the holidays because they've probably indulged in far too much rubbish themselves. If you're at a party, people dive into the vegetables dip rather than chips because we all generally want to eat healthily. I always see the vegetable and dip platter go down quicker than any other snack food.

One good thing about the holidays is most of the food is centered around a protein. Turkey for Thanksgiving, and in my house, turkey, duck or ham for Christmas. These are GO proteins you can fill up on until you're satisfied. Just have smaller portions of the carb dishes and you'll be fine.

Also, a few bites of pumpkin pie are not going to be the end of the world, so enjoy it while it's there.

"What about alcohol on Vacation? You don't advocate having more than one drink a day at the most, and definitely no cocktails, so what if I want a few drinks?"

My answer is always the same as eating. Have fun but don't go crazy. I know this seems like a mixed message compared to the nutrition plan and everything else I've said about balancing the Five Pillars. But I firmly believe if you are to have more control over food choices and food impulses, you need to know that you can be flexible if you are also responsible. Do I advocate having ten beers in a day on vacation? Absolutely not. Do I think a few cocktails around the pool while you're relaxing can have a positive effect on your body, mind, and blood? Yes, I do.

If you can learn that a little of what you like now and then can be beneficial, then you'll find it so much easier to stay on your plan for longer. This flexibility will give you more significant long-term benefits to your blood and health. Now, would I be disappointed if you brought these habits back with you and continued to have more off-plan food and drink? Absolutely, but vacations are a place for recharging your batteries, relaxing and de-stressing, and this plays a significant role in cleansing your blood.

So yes, go away and have fun. Don't go crazy with your choices and come back ready to get back on plan with renewed motivation.

You've Got This!

I hope by now you have a clear and realistic idea of what's going on in your body and you've created your own realistic roadmap on how to move forward. From working with countless people who started in the same position as you I just want you to know there is light at the end of the tunnel. And that tunnel is a lot shorter than you think.

I want to thank you for giving me the opportunity to share my knowledge with you and from here on in, you are the Captain of your destiny and I have every faith that you'll be fine. Just follow the guide, be kind to yourself, don't set your expectations too high, be flexible, and take each meal at a time. Oh, and always remember: Progress not perfection!

Before I sign off, I want to wish you well and I'll leave you with this quote from Ralph Waldo Emerson which sums up what it means to go through this process to cleanse your blood.

"For everything you have missed, you have gained something else, and for everything you gain, you lose something else."

Be well and have a happy long life.

Drew

References

1. Lavery JA, Friedman AM, Keyes KM, Wright JD, Ananth CV. Gestational diabetes in the United States: temporal changes in prevalence rates between 1979 and 2010. BJOG 2017;124:804–813.
2. Suckale J, Solimena M (2008). Pancreas islets in metabolic signaling-focus on the beta-cell. [Frontiers in Bioscience 13, 7156-7171, May 1, 2008.
3. Centers for Disease Control and Prevention. National Diabetes Statistics Report, 2017. Atlanta, GA: Centers for Disease Control and Prevention, US Department of Health and Human Services; 2017.
4. Alberti K. G. M. M., Eckel R. H., Grundy S. M., et al., "Harmonizing the metabolic syndrome: a joint interim statement of the international diabetes federation task force on epidemiology and prevention; National heart, lung, and blood institute; American heart association; World heart federation; International atherosclerosis society; And international association for the study of obesity," Circulation, vol. 120, no. 16, pp. 1640–1645, 2009.
5. Mozumdar A, Liguori G. Persistent increase of prevalence of metabolic syndrome among US adults: NHANES III to NHANES 1999-2006. Diabetes Care. 2011;34(1):216-219.
6. Park Y, Zhu S, Palaniappan L, Heshka S, Carnethon MR, Heymsfield SB. The Metabolic Syndrome Prevalence and Associated Risk Factor Findings in the US Population From the Third National Health and Nutrition Examination Survey, 1988-1994. Arch Intern Med. 2003;163(4):427–436. doi:10.1001/archinte.163.4.427.
7. Wagenknecht LE, Mayer EJ, Rewers M, et al. The Insulin Resistance Atherosclerosis Study (IRAS) objectives, design, and recruitment results. Ann Epidemiol. 1995;5:464-472.
8. Wing RR, Koeske R, Epstein LH, Nowalk MP, Gooding W, Becker D. Long-term effects of modest weight loss in type II diabetic patients. Arch Intern Med. 1987;147:1749-1753.
9. Stevens VJ, Obarzanek E, Cook NR, Lee I, Appel LJ, Smith West D, et al. Long-Term Weight Loss and Changes in Blood Pressure: Results of the Trials of Hypertension Prevention, Phase II. Ann Intern Med. ;134:1–11. doi: 10.7326/0003-4819-134-1-200101020-00007.
10. Chaoyang Li, Earl S. Ford, Benyi Li, Wayne H. Giles, Simin Liu. Association of Testosterone and Sex Hormone–Binding Globulin With Metabolic Syndrome and Insulin Resistance in Men Diabetes Care Jul 2010, 33 (7) 1618-1624; DOI: 10.2337/dc09-1788.
11. Eric L. Ding, Sc.D., Yiqing Song, M.D. et al. Sex Hormone–Binding Globulin and Risk of Type 2 Diabetes in Women and Men. N Engl J Med 2009; 361:1152-1163 DOI: 10.1056/NEJMoa0804381.
12. SM, Hryb DJ, Nakhla AM, Romas NA, Rosner W. Sex hormone-binding globulin is synthesized in target cells. J Endocrinol 2002;175:113-120.

13. Ding EL, Song Y, Malik VS, Liu S. Sex differences of endogenous sex hormones and risk of type 2 diabetes: a systematic review and meta-analysis. JAMA 2006;295:1288-1299.
14. Lindstedt G, Lundberg PA, Lapidus L, Lundgren H, Bengtsson C, Bjorntorp P. Low sex-hormone-binding globulin concentration as independent risk factor for development of NIDDM: 12-yr follow-up of population study of women in Gothenburg, Sweden. Diabetes 1991;40:123-128.
15. Dunning B. E., Gerich J. E. (2007). The role of alpha-cell dysregulation in fasting and postprandial hyperglycemia in type 2 diabetes and therapeutic implications. Endocr. Rev. 8, 253–283 10.1210/er.2006-0026.
16. Quesada I., Tudurí E., Ripoll C., Nadal A. (2008). Physiology of the pancreatic alpha-cell and glucagon secretion: role in glucose homeostasis and diabetes. J. Endocrinol. 199, 5–19 10.1677/JOE-08-0290.
17. Gil-Campos M, et al. "Ghrelin: a hormone regulating food intake and energy homeostasis." The British Journal of Nutrition August 2006.
18. Andrews ZB, Erion DM, Beiler R, Choi CS, Shulman GI, Horvath TL. Uncoupling Protein-2 Decreases the Lipogenic Actions of Ghrelin. Endocrinology. 2010;151:2078–86.
19. Sun Y, Asnicar M, Saha PK, et al. Ablation of ghrelin improves the diabetic but not obese phenotype of ob/ob mice. Cell metabolism. 2006;3:379–86.
20. Chacko SK, Haymond MW, Sun Y, et al. Effect of ghrelin on glucose regulation in mice. Am J Physiol Endocrinol Metab. 2012;302:E1055–62.
21. Müller TD, Nogueiras R, Andermann ML, et al. Ghrelin. Molecular Metabolism. 2015;4(6):437-460. doi:10.1016/j.molmet.2015.03.005.
22. Chuang JC, Sakata I, Kohno D, Perello M, Osborne-Lawrence S, et al. Ghrelin Directly Stimulates Glucagon Secretion from Pancreatic α-Cells. Mol Endocrinol. 2011 September; 25(9): 1600–1611.
23. Chuang JC, Sakata I, Kohno D, et al. Ghrelin directly stimulates glucagon secretion from pancreatic alpha-cells. Mol Endocrinol. 2011;25:1600–11.
24. Mao Y, Tokudome T, Otani K, et al. Excessive sympathoactivation and deteriorated heart function after myocardial infarction in male ghrelin knockout mice. Endocrinology. 2013;154:1854–63.
25. Gagnon J, Sheppard E, Anini Y. Metformin directly inhibits ghrelin secretion through AMP-activated protein kinase in rat primary gastric cells. Diabetes, obesity & metabolism. 2013;15:276–9.
26. Considine RV, Sinha MK, Heiman ML et al. Serum immunoreactive-leptin concentrations in normal-weight and obese humans. N Engl J Med 1996;334:292–295.
27. Wauters M; Considine RV; Yudkin, JS; Peiffer, F; De Leeuw, I; Van Gaal, LF; (2003) Leptin levels in type 2 diabetes: associations with measures of insulin resistance and insulin secretion. Horm Metab Res , 35 (2) pp. 92-96.
28. Ahima RS, Prabakaran D, Mantzoros C et al. Role of leptin in the neuroendocrine response to fasting. Nature 1996;382:250–252.
29. Hua X, Carvalho N, Tew M, Huang ES, Herman WH, Clarke P. Expenditures and Prices of Antihyperglycemic Medications in the United States: 2002-2013. JAMA. 2016;315(13):1400–1402. doi:10.1001/jama.2016.0126.
30. Wing R.R (1999). Physical activity in the treatment of the adulthood overweight and obesity: current evidence and research issues. Med Sci Sports Exerc. 1999 Nov;31(11 Suppl):S547-52.

31. Moran C, Beare R, Phan TG, Bruce D.G, Callisaya ML, Srikanth V. Type 2 diabetes mellitus and biomarkers of neurodegeneration. Neurology Sep 2015, 10.1212/WNL.0000000000001982; DOI: 10.1212/WNL.0000000000001982.
32. Suzanne M, Tong M. Brain metabolic dysfunction at the core of Alzheimer's disease Biochem. Pharmacol., 88 (2014), pp.548-559.
33. McNay EC, Recknagel AK. Brain insulin signaling: a key component of cognitive processes and a potential basis for cognitive impairment in type 2 diabetes. Neurobiol Learn Mem. 2011 October; 96(3): 432–442.
34. Raffaitin C, Gin H, Empana J-P, et al. Metabolic Syndrome and Risk for Incident Alzheimer's Disease or Vascular Dementia: The Three-City Study. Diabetes Care. 2009;32(1):169-174. doi:10.2337/dc08-0272.
35. Ismail Y, Ismail AA, Ismail AA. The underestimated problem of using serum magnesium measurements to exclude magnesium deficiency in adults; a health warning is needed for "normal" results. Clin Chem Lab Med. 2010 Mar; 48(3):323-7.
36. Evidence-Based Recommendations for Optimal Dietary Protein Intake in Older People: A Position Paper From the PROT-AGE Study Group Bauer, Jürgen et al. Journal of the American Medical Directors Association, Volume 14, Issue 8, 542 – 559.
37. Layman DK, Anthony TG, Rasmussen BB, Adams SH, Lynch CJ, Brinkworth GD, Davis TA. 2015. Defining meal requirements for protein to optimize metabolic roles of amino acids. Am. J. Clin. Nutr. **101**(6): 1330S-1338S.
38. Phillips SM, Chevalier S, Leidy HJ. 2016. Protein "requirements" beyond the RDA: implications for optimizing health. Applied Physiology, Nutrition, and Metabolism, 2016, 41:565-572.
39. de Souza RJ, Mente A, Maroleanu A, et al. Intake of saturated and trans unsaturated fatty acids and risk of all cause mortality, cardiovascular disease, and type 2 diabetes: systematic review and meta-analysis of observational studies. BMJ 2015;351:h3978.
40. Malhotra A, Redberg RF, Meier P. Saturated fat does not clog the arteries: coronary heart disease is a chronic inflammatory condition, the risk of which can be effectively reduced from healthy lifestyle interventions. Br J Sports Med.
41. Libby P. Inflammation and cardiovascular disease mechanisms. Am J Clin Nutr. 2006 Feb;83(2):456S-460S.
42. Riaz A. Memon, Ilona Staprans, Mustafa Noor et al. Infection and Inflammation Induce LDL Oxidation In Vivo. Arteriosclerosis, Thrombosis, and Vascular Biology. 2000;20:1536-1542.
43. Wolever TMS, Piekarz A, Hollands R, Younker K. Sugar Alcohols and Diabetes:A Review. Canadian Journal of Diabetes. 2002;26(4):356-362.
44. Ross R, Janssen I. (2001). Physical activity, total and regional obesity: dose-response considerations. Med Sci Sports Exerc. 2001 Jun;33(6 Suppl):S521-7; discussion S528-9.
45. Kerns, J. C., Guo, J., Fothergill, E., Howard, L., Knuth, N. D., Brychta, R., Chen, K. Y., Skarulis, M. C., Walter, P. J. and Hall, K. D. (2017), Increased Physical Activity Associated with Less Weight Regain Six Years After "The Biggest Loser" Competition. Obesity, 25: 1838–1843. doi:10.1002/oby.21986.
46. Mourier A, Gautier JF, De Kerviler E, Bigard AX, Villette JM, Garnier JP, Duvallet A, Guezennec CY, Cathelineau G: Mobilization of visceral adipose tissue related to the improvement in insulin sensitivity in response to physical training in NIDDM: effects of branched-chain amino acid supplements. Diabetes Care 20:385–391, 1997.

47. Ruderman NB, Ganda OP, Johansen K: The effect of physical training on glucose tolerance and plasma lipids in maturity-onset diabetes. Diabetes 28(Suppl. 1):S89–S92, 1979.
48. Baldi JC, Snowling N: Resistance training improves glycaemic control in obese type 2 diabetic men. Int J Sports Med 24:419–423, 2003.
49. Castaneda C, Layne JE, Munoz-Orians L, Gordon PL, Walsmith J, Foldvari M, Roubenoff R, Tucker KL, Nelson ME: A randomized controlled trial of resistance exercise training to improve glycemic control in older adults with type 2 diabetes. Diabetes Care 25:2335–2341, 2002.
50. Jelleyman C, Yates T, O'Donovan G, et al. The effects of high-intensity interval training on glucose regulation and insulin resistance: a meta-analysis. Obes Rev 2015;16:942–961.
51. Little JP, Gillen JB, Percival ME, et al. Low-volume high-intensity interval training reduces hyperglycemia and increases muscle mitochondrial capacity in patients with type 2 diabetes. J Appl Physiol (1985) 2011;111:1554–1560.
52. Arciero PJ, Ormsbee MJ, Gentile CL, Nindl BC, Brestoff JR, Ruby M. Increased protein intake and meal frequency reduces abdominal fat during energy balance and energy deficit. Obesity (Silver Spring). 2013 Jul;21(7):1357-66. doi: 10.1002/oby.20296. Epub 2013 May 23.
53. The cost of organic food. https://www.consumerreports.org/cro/news/2015/03/cost-of-organic-food/index.htm
54. The National List of Allowed and Prohibited Substances in organic agriculture. https://bit.ly/2pGPz63 (author shortened link).
55. Are Organic Foods Safer or Healthier Than Conventional Alternatives? A Systematic Review. Crystal Smith-Spangler, MD, MS; Margaret L. Brandeau, Ph.D. et al. Ann Intern Med. 2012;157.
56. Mondelaers, K., Aertsens, J., Van Huylenbroeck, G., 2009. A meta-analysis of the differences in environmental impacts between organic and conventional farming. British Food Journal 111, 1098e1119.
57. Epstein SS. Unlabeled Milk from Cows Treated with Biosynthetic Growth Hormones: A Case of Regulatory Abdication. International Journal of Health Services Vol 26, Issue 1, pp. 173 – 185.
58. FDA: Guidance for Industry: Voluntary Labeling Indicating Whether Foods Have or Have Not Been Derived from Genetically Engineered Plants. https://bit.ly/2GxoRtb (author shortened link).
59. FDA: Labeling of Foods Derived From Genetically Engineered Plants. https://bit.ly/2GxoRtb (author shortened link).
60. Tortora, R., Capone, P., De Stefano, G., Imperatore, N., Gerbino, N., Donetto, S., Monaco, V., Caporaso, N. and Rispo, A. (2015), Metabolic syndrome in patients with coeliac disease on a gluten-free diet. Aliment Pharmacol Ther, 41: 352-359. doi:10.1111/apt.13062.
61. Jenkins DJ, Kendall CW, Augustin LS, Martini MC, Axelsen M, Faulkner D, Vidgen E, Parker T, Lau H, et al. Effect of wheat bran on glycemic control and risk factors for cardiovascular disease in type 2 diabetes. Diabetes Care. 2002; 25:1522–8.
62. Leidy HJ, Bales-Voelker LI, Harris CT. A protein-rich beverage consumed as a breakfast meal leads to weaker appetitive and dietary responses v. a protein-rich solid breakfast meal in adolescents. Br J Nutr. 2011 Jul;106(1):37-41. doi: 10.1017/S0007114511000122. Epub 2011 Feb 15.

63. Bhattacharyya S, Borthakur A, Dudeja PK, Tobacman JK, "Carrageenan induces interleukin-8 production through distinct Bcl10 pathway in normal human colonic epithelial cells," The American Journal of Physiology, vol. 292, no. 3, pp. G829–G838, 2007.
64. Bhattacharyya S, Gill R, Mei LC, et al., "Toll-like receptor 4 mediates induction of the Bcl10-NFκB-interleukin-8 inflammatory pathway by carrageenan in human intestinal epithelial cells," The Journal of Biological Chemistry, vol. 283, no. 16, pp. 10550–10558, 2008.
65. Tobacman JK, "Review of harmful gastrointestinal effects of carrageenan in animal experiments," Environmental Health Perspectives, vol. 109, no. 10, pp. 983–994, 2001.
66. IARC Working Group on the Evaluation of the Carcinogenic Risk of Chemicals to Humans, "Carrageenan," IARC Monographs on the Evaluation of Carcinogenic Risks to Humans, vol. 31, pp. 79–94, 1983.
67. Farshchi HR, Taylor MA, Macdonald IA. Beneficial metabolic effects of regular meal frequency on dietary thermogenesis, insulin sensitivity, and fasting lipid profiles in healthy obese women. Am J Clin Nutr 2005;81:16–24.
68. Farshchi HR, Taylor MA, Macdonald IA. Deleterious effects of omitting breakfast on insulin sensitivity and fasting lipid profiles in healthy lean women. Am J Clin Nutr 2005;81:388–396.
69. Fabry P, Fodor J, Hejl Z, Geizerova H, Balcarova O. Meal frequency and ischaemic heart disease. Lancet 1968;2:190–191.
70. Jenkins DJ, Wolever TM, Vuksan V et al. Nibbling versus gorging metabolic advantages of increased meal frequency. N Engl J Med 1989;321:929–934.
71. Sierra-Johnson, J., Undén, A. L., Linestrand, M., Rosell, M., Sjogren, P., Kolak, M., ... & Hellénius, M. L. (2008). Eating meals irregularly: a novel environmental risk factor for the metabolic syndrome. Obesity, 16(6), 1302-1307.
72. Leidy HJ, Ortinau LC, Douglas SM, Hoertel HA. Am J Clin Nutr. 2013 Apr; 97(4):677-88. Epub 2013 Feb 27.
73. Leidy HJ, Hoertel HA, Douglas SM, Higgins KA, Shafer RS. Obesity (Silver Spring). 2015 Sep; 23(9):1761-4. Epub 2015 Aug 4.
74. Leidy HJ, Racki E. The addition of a protein-rich breakfast and its effects on acute appetite control and food intake in "breakfast-skipping" adolescents. International journal of obesity (2005). 2010;34(7):1125-1133. doi:10.1038/ijo.2010.3.
75. University of Sydney. (2016, July 12). Why artificial sweeteners can increase appetite. *ScienceDaily*. Retrieved March 20, 2018.
76. Qiao-Ping Wang, Yong Qi Lin, Lei Zhang, Yana A. Wilson, Lisa J. Oyston, James Cotterell, Yue Qi, Thang M. Khuong, Noman Bakhshi, Yoann Planchenault, Duncan T. Browman, Man Tat Lau, Tiffany A. Cole, Adam C.N. Wong, Stephen J. Simpson, Adam R. Cole, Josef M. Penninger, Herbert Herzog, G. Gregory Neely. Sucralose Promotes Food Intake through NPY and a Neuronal Fasting Response. Cell Metabolism, 2016; 24 (1): 75 DOI: 10.1016/j.cmet.2016.06.010.
77. Kiage JN, Merrill PD, Robinson CJ, Cao Y, Malik TA, Hundley BC, et al. Intake of *trans* fat and all-cause mortality in the Reasons for Geographical and Racial Differences in Stroke (REGARDS) cohort, *The American Journal of Clinical Nutrition*, Volume 97, Issue 5, 1 May 2013, Pages 1121–1128.
78. Moeller SM, Parekh N, Tinker L, et al. Associations Between Intermediate Age-Related Macular Degeneration and Lutein and Zeaxanthin in the Carotenoids in

Age-Related Eye Disease Study (CAREDS)Ancillary Study of the Women's Health Initiative. *Arch Ophthalmol.* 2006;124(8):1151–1162. doi:10.1001/archopht.124.8.1151.
79. Semba RD, Dagnelie D. Are lutein and zeaxanthin conditionally essential nutrients for eye health? Medical Hypotheses (2003) 61(4), 465–472. doi:10.1016/S0306-9877(03)00198-1.
80. IMS Institute for Healthcare Informatics. National Prescription Audit December 2012. Available from www.imshealth.com. Accessed 3 May 2017.
81. Hajnal A, Norgren R. Taste pathways that mediate accumbens dopamine release by sapid sucrose. Physiol Behav 2005;84:363–369. [PubMed: 15763573].
82. Roitman MF, Stuber GD, Phillips PEM, Wightman RM, Carelli RM. Dopamine operates as a subsecond modulator of food seeking. J Neurosci 2004;24:1265–1271. [PubMed: 14960596].
83. Berridge KC. 'Liking' and 'wanting' food rewards: Brain substrates and roles in eating disorders. Physiol Behav. 2009 July 14; 97(5): 537–550.
84. Simpson SJ, Raubenheimer D. Obesity: the protein leverage hypothesis. Obes Rev 2005; 6:133–42.
85. Martens EA, Lemmens S, Westerterp-Plantenga M. Protein leverage affects energy intake of high-protein diets in humans. Am J Clin Nutr 2013; 97:86–93.
86. Prochaska, J. O., DiClemente, C. C., & Norcross, J. C. (1992). In search of how people change: Applications to addictive behaviors. Am Psychol, 47, 1102–1114.
87. Hicks, R. A., McTighe, S., & Juarez, M. (1986). Sleep duration and eating behaviors in college students. Perceptual and Motor Skills, Vol 62, Issue 1, pp. 209 - 210.
88. Wells TT, Cruess DG. Effects of partial sleep deprivation on food consumption and food choice. Psychology and Health, February 2006, 21(1): 79–86.
89. Hamburg NM, McMackin CJ, Huang AL, et al. Physical Inactivity Rapidly Induces Insulin Resistance and Microvascular Dysfunction in Healthy Volunteers. Arteriosclerosis, Thrombosis, and Vascular Biology. 2007;27:2650-2656.
90. Stephens BR, et al. Effects of 1 day of inactivity on insulin action in healthy men and women: interaction with energy intake. Metabolism - Clinical and Experimental, July 2011, Volume 60, Issue 7, 941 – 949.
91. Francis ME, Pennebaker JW. Putting Stress into Words: The Impact of Writing on Physiological, Absentee, and Self-Reported Emotional Well-Being Measures. American Journal of Health Promotion Vol 6, Issue 4, pp. 280 – 287. First Published March 1, 1992.
92. Hiemstra, R. (2001), Uses and benefits of journal writing. New Directions for Adult and Continuing Education, 2001: 19–26. doi:10.1002/ace.17.
93. Yamanouchi K, Shinozaki T, Chikada K, et al. Daily Walking Combined With Diet Therapy Is a Useful Means for Obese NIDDM Patients Not Only to Reduce Body Weight But Also to Improve Insulin Sensitivity. Diabetes Care Jun 1995, 18 (6) 775-778; DOI: 10.2337/diacare.18.6.775.
94. Rong-fang Hu, Xiao-ying Jiang, Yi-ming Zeng, Xiao-yang Chen and You-hua Zhang. Effects of earplugs and eye masks on nocturnal sleep, melatonin and cortisol in a simulated intensive care unit environment. Critical Care201014:R66. https://doi.org/10.1186/cc8965

About The Author

Drew Coster is a Psychotherapist with a Masters in Rational, Emotive and Cognitive Behavior Therapy from Goldsmiths, University of London. Drew has worked as a therapist for nearly two decades in a wide range of ways including in a Psychiatric Hospital, a college, Silicon Valley Startups, and Private Practice. He occasionally works with people remotely through his website drewcoster.com while continuing his passion of writing.

Printed in Great Britain
by Amazon